Augmentation Fillers

FILLER TECHNIQUES are the most widely used surgical procedures in cosmetic surgery, as they are the best method of reducing wrinkles on a long-term basis. For years, dermatologists have known that water-binding soft tissue fillers can replace the loss of collagen, elastin, and hyaluronic acid from the skin. Because filler formulas and application techniques are constantly updated and reevaluated, the dermatologist and cosmetic surgeon need a quick reference on the subject. This new text, edited by world-renowned dermatologist Dr. Neil S. Sadick, covers all the main aspects of soft tissue filler techniques. Subjects covered include choosing and applying fillers; short-, intermediate-, and long-acting fillers; and combination approaches, as well as anesthetic considerations, equipment and patient positioning, operative procedures, potential complications, and postoperative evaluation.

Neil S. Sadick, MD, FAAD, FAACS, FACP, FACPh, is in private practice in dermatology at Sadick Dermatology and Aesthetic Surgery, located in New York City and Great Neck, New York. Dr. Sadick is Clinical Professor of Dermatology at Weill Cornell Medical College and Associate Attending Physician in the Division of Dermatology at North Shore University Hospital. Dr. Sadick has written more than 500 articles and ten books on cosmetic dermatology.

AUGMENTATION FILLERS

Edited by

Neil S. Sadick

Weill Cornell Medical College, New York, New York

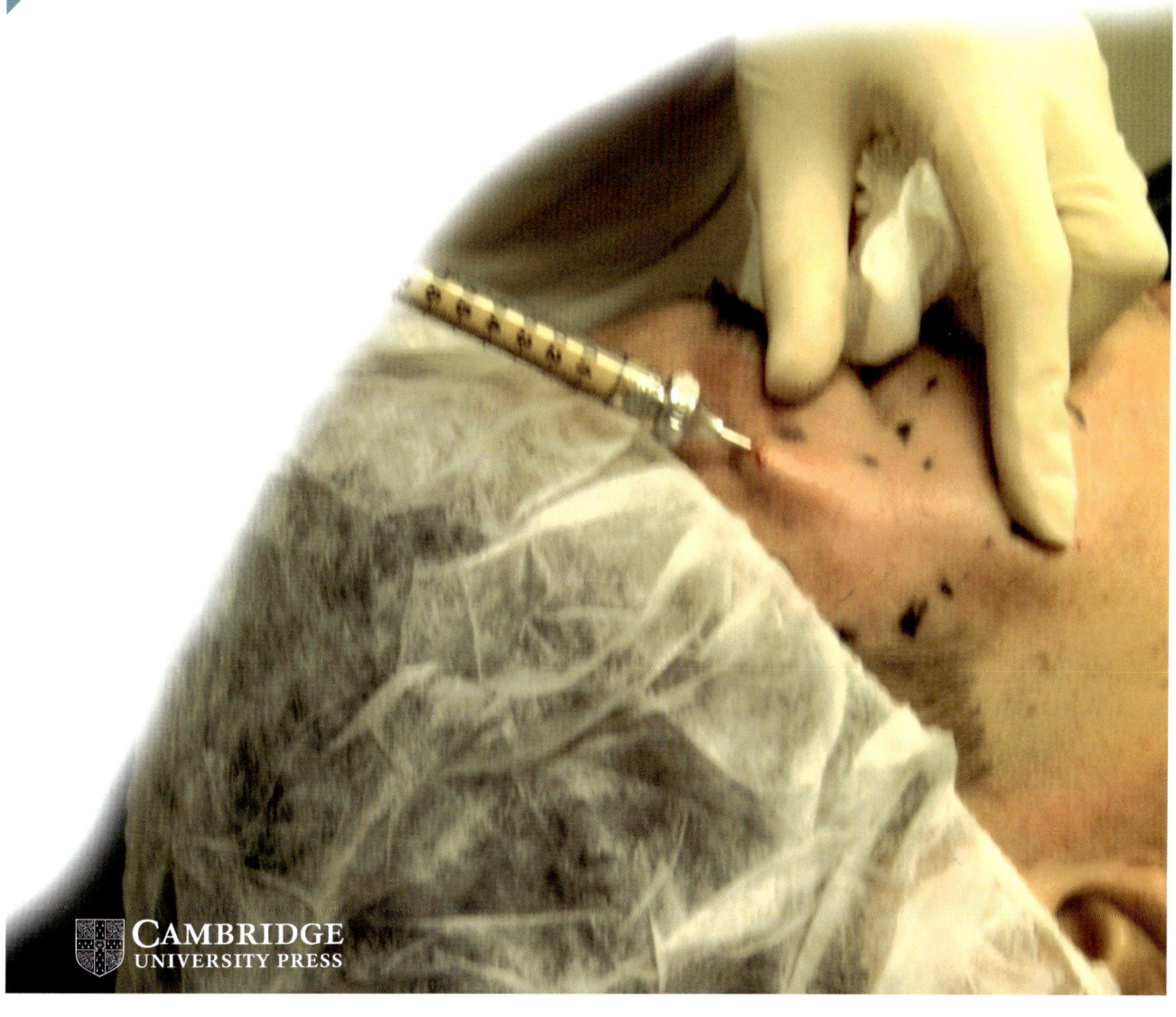

CAMBRIDGE
UNIVERSITY PRESS

CAMBRIDGE UNIVERSITY PRESS
Cambridge, New York, Melbourne, Madrid, Cape Town, Singapore,
São Paulo, Delhi, Dubai, Tokyo

Cambridge University Press
32 Avenue of the Americas, New York, NY 10013-2473, USA

www.cambridge.org
Information on this title: www.cambridge.org/9780521881128

© Cambridge University Press 2010

First published 2010

Printed in China by Everbest

A catalog record for this publication is available from the British Library.

Library of Congress Cataloging in Publication Data

Augmentation fillers / edited by Neil S. Sadick.
p. ; cm.
Includes bibliographical references and index.
ISBN 978-0-521-88112-8 (hardback)
1. Tissue expansion. 2. Fillers (Materials) 3. Surgery, Plastic. I. Sadick, Neil S. [DNLM: 1. Cosmetic Techniques.
2. Face–surgery. 3. Biopolymers–therapeutic use. 4. Dermatologic Agents–therapeutic use.
5. Injections, Subcutaneous. 6. Tissue Expansion–methods. WE 705 A919 2009]

RD119.5.T57A94 2009
617.9′52–dc22   2009027825

ISBN 978-0-521-88112-8 Hardback

Contents

List of Contributors

Robert Anolik, MD
Allergy and Immunology
Blue Bell, Pennsylvania

Sumit Bapna, MD
Dermatology (Private Practice)
San Francisco, California, and
Division of Facial Plastic Surgery
Department of Otolaryngology
University of California, San Francisco
San Francisco, California

Joel L. Cohen, MD
Dermatology (Private Practice)
Englewood, Colorado

Steven R. Cohen, MD, FACS
Plastic Surgery
    (Private Practice)
La Jolla, California, and
Division of Plastic Surgery
University of California, San Diego
San Diego, California

Lisa M. Donofrio, MD
Dermatology (Private Practice)
New Haven, Connecticut

Ellen Gendler, MD
Dermatology (Private Practice)
New York, New York, and
Department of Dermatology

New York University School of Medicine
New York, New York

David J. Goldberg, MD
Department of Dermatology
Mount Sinai School of Medicine
New York, New York

Harriet Lin Hall, ARNP
Dermatology (Private Practice)
Bradenton, Florida

C. William Hanke, MD, MPH, FACP
Dermatology (Private Practice)
Indianapolis, Indiana

Ranella J. Hirsch, MD
Dermatology (Private Practice)
Cambridge, Massachusetts, and
President, American Society
    of Cosmetic Surgery and Aesthetic Surgery

Derek Jones, MD
Dermatology (Private Practice)
Beverly Hills, California, and
Department of Medicine
University of California, Los Angeles
Los Angeles, California

Cheryl Karcher, MD
Dermatology (Private Practice)
New York, New York

Mary P. Lupo, MD, FAAD
Dermatology (Private Practice)
New Orleans, Louisiana, and
Past President,
    Women's Dermatologic Society

Corey S. Maas, MD
Dermatology
    (Private Practice)
San Francisco, California, and
Division of Facial Plastic Surgery
Department of Otolaryngology
University of California, San Francisco
San Francisco, California

Gary D. Monheit, MD
Dermatology
    (Private Practice)
Birmingham, Alabama, and
Department of Dermatology
University of Alabama
    at Birmingham
Birmingham, Alabama

Andrew A. Nelson, MD
Department of Dermatology
Harvard Medical School
Boston, Massachusetts

Chad Prather, MD
Dermatology (Private Practice)
Baton Rouge, Louisiana

Kelley Pagliai Redbord, MD
Dermatology (Private Practice)
Indianapolis, Indiana

Deborshi Roy, MD
Dermatology (Private Practice)
New York, New York

Mark G. Rubin, MD
Dermatology (Private Practice)
Beverly Hills, California, and
Division of Dermatology
University of California, San Diego
San Diego, California

Neil S. Sadick, MD
Dermatology (Private Practice)
New York, New York, and
Department of Dermatology
New York Presbyterian-Weill Cornell
    Medical College
New York, New York, and
President, Cosmetic Surgery Foundation

Papri Sarkar, MD
Department of Dermatology
Brigham and Women's Hospital
Boston, Massachusetts

Susan H. Weinkle, MD
Dermatology (Private Practice)
Bradenton, Florida

Chapter 1

APPLICATION OF FILLERS

by

Deborshi Roy, MD

INTRODUCTION

In the last five years, there has been an increased demand in the number of fillers available in the market. This corresponds with the increased demand for less-invasive procedures among consumers. The result is a wide array of choices for the patient and injector to address almost any type of problem. In this chapter, we outline the various applications of fillers throughout the body.

BACKGROUND

The ideal injectable filler remains elusive to this day. The properties we look for in an ideal injectable filler include safety, ease of use, consistency of results, and longevity of results.

Liquid silicone was the first filler available to treat contour defects, scars, and rhytids of the face. It was widely used for two decades until concerns about long-term safety caused it to fall out of favor.[1,2] Several years ago, a new liquid silicone product was cleared by the FDA and has been used in an "off-label" fashion for cosmetic enhancement of the face. Liquid silicone is a permanent filler.

Bovine collagen was the second available injectable filler and was widely used with a very low incidence of complications.[3] Allergy testing of the skin was necessary with Zyderm and Zyplast. These products lasted for a few months after injection, requiring frequent administration. Over the years, collagen-based products have evolved. Cosmoderm and Cosmoplast (human collagen) eliminated the need for skin testing. Evolence (porcine collagen) is cross-linked, giving it a longer-lasting quality, and it does not require skin testing.

Autologous fat transfer techniques were introduced around the same time as bovine collagen. The safety of an autologous filler cannot be matched by anything synthetic. However, there is an increased morbidity associated with a more invasive type of procedure. Consistent, reproducible results are also an obstacle for some practitioners.

Hyaluronic acid fillers are among the pack of the latest, most widely used nonsurgical cosmetic treatments. Hyaluronic acid products can be derived from animal sources or from bacterial fermentation (see Table 1.1). The various preparations currently available differ in cross-linking and concentration of hyaluronic acid in the carrier vehicle. Although the products are all similar, there are subtle differences that lead each injector to have his or her own

TABLE 1.1. Various Hyaluronic Acid Injectable Filler Preparations

Juvederm Ultra Juvederm Ultraplus	Nonanimal Stabilized Hyaluronic Acid (NASHA)
Restylane Perlane Elevess Hylaform	NASHA NASHA + Lidocaine Animal hyaluronic acid

preference. Most hyaluronic acid fillers last from four to six months.

Radiesse comprises microspheres of calcium hydroxylapatite suspended in a matrix composed of water, glycerin, and sodium carboxymethylcellulose. This is a bulkier product than those previously mentioned, and it is injected into a deeper plane. The unique viscosity and elasticity of the material make it possible to mold the implant for several minutes after injection, minimizing irregularities in contour. Unlike the previous products, Radiesse has been shown to stimulate new collagen growth in the injected areas. It lasts from eight to twelve months.

Sculptra is a suspension of poly-L-lactic acid in water. Unlike the previously mentioned products, it is not used in a single injection session. To obtain optimal results, multiple injection sessions several weeks apart must be utilized. This product can also induce new collagen growth and has been clinically shown to increase dermal thickness over time, with results lasting for several years.

Artefill is a combination of polymethylmethacrylate (PMMA) spheres and bovine collagen. This product requires skin testing and can last for several years as the bovine collagen is replaced by autologous neo-collagen over time since the PMMA spheres provide a permanent platform.

BASIC APPROACHES TO INJECTABLE FILLERS

There are two main approaches when it comes to using any type of injectable filler. The first is the microscopic approach – zooming in and concentrating on specific lines, wrinkles, furrows, or scars. The second approach is the macroscopic – pulling back and reconstituting lost volume. It is important to keep both approaches in mind when addressing any given situation since most problems are multifactorial and require a thorough evaluation for effective treatment. Injectable fillers are often combined with other treatment modalities to achieve a global rejuvenation of the skin and soft tissue.

BASIC INJECTION TECHNIQUES

There are several injection techniques, and each injector has his or her favorite. There are some situations where one technique is preferred over the others due to anatomic constraints or the depth of injection required. The main techniques are serial puncture, linear threading, cross-hatching, fanning, and depot (see Figure 1.1). Although most injectors prefer using transcutaneous injection techniques, there are several transoral injection techniques described.

ANATOMICAL CONSIDERATIONS

When addressing the face, we like to divide it into upper, middle, and lower thirds. Of course, all three must be balanced to achieve a harmonious, pleasing appearance.

The upper third of the face includes the forehead, glabella, and periorbital areas. Here, the synergistic use of botulinum toxin combined with injectable fillers for the treatment of dynamic rhytids can achieve better results than a single-modality treatment.[4]

Posttraumatic or iatrogenic defects of the forehead and temporal areas can be treated with fillers with great success. In periorbital rejuvenation, volume replacement is the key. Temporal lipoatrophy can be reversed with injectable fillers. Mild brow ptosis can be alleviated with a combination of botulinum toxin and volume augmentation. The naso-jugal crease or

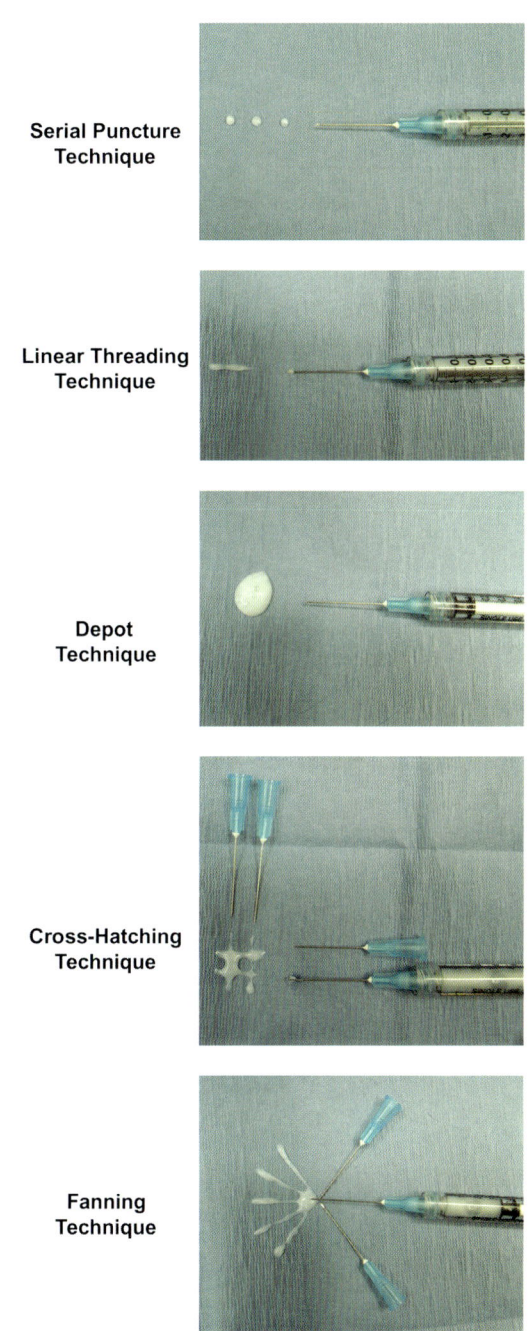

Serial Puncture
Technique

Linear Threading
Technique

Depot
Technique

Cross-Hatching
Technique

Fanning
Technique

FIG. 1.1. Various injection techniques: serial puncture, linear threading, depot, cross-hatching, and fanning.

"tear trough" deformity can be treated with careful injection of filler into this area.

The midface is the most popular area for use of injectable fillers. Soft tissue volume loss is an integral part of the aging process. The nasolabial folds are the most commonly treated area of the face. All of the available injectable fillers have been used in this area with a great deal of success. Treatment of malar and submalar volume loss is also very common when dealing with HIV-associated facial lipoatrophy.[5]

Treatment of posttraumatic or congenital defects of the nose is another area of the midface where injectable fillers can be used to avoid the need for surgical intervention. Scars of the face (especially those due to acne) are most commonly treated in the midface, in the mid-to-lateral cheek areas.

In the lower face, treatment of perioral rhytids is the most common application of injectable fillers. Volume enhancement of the lips is also very common. Other areas that are treated include the jawline and chin, especially the prejowl sulcus.

Off-face use of fillers has grown considerably in the last few years. One of the most common areas of use off the face is for rejuvenation of the hands. Volume replacement of the dorsal hands can be achieved with fillers alone or fillers combined with light-based modalities.

Fillers have also been widely used in postreconstructive nipple enhancement and postliposuction defects anywhere on the body.

CONCLUSION

There are a myriad of choices when it comes to injectable fillers. The most important aspect of deciding which filler to choose for any particular treatment is the clinical evaluation of the patient. Other considerations, such as the anatomical area being treated, the depth of the injection, and the desired duration of results, can also influence the choice of filler used. Fillers can also be combined with surgical and nonsurgical treatment modalities. With the appropriate assessment of the patient's concerns, several options can be presented, and an informed decision can be made.

REFERENCES

1. Aronsohn RB: A 22-year experience with the use of silicone injections. *American Journal of Cosmetic Surgery* **1**:21–28, 1984

2. Pearl RM, Laub DR, Kaplan EN: Complications following silicone injections for augmentation of the contours of the face. *Plastic and Reconstructive Surgery* **61**:888–891, 1978

3. Cooperman LS, Mackinnon V, Bechler G, Pharriss B: Injectable collagen: a six-year clinical investigation. *Aesthetic Plastic Surgery* **79**:581–594, 1987

4. Carruthers J, Carruthers A: A prospective, randomized, parallel group study analyzing the effect of botulinum toxin A and non-animal sourced hyaluronic acid. *Dermatologic Surgery* Aug;**29**(8):802–809, 2003

5. Silvers SL, Eviatar JA, Echavez MI, Pappas AL: Prospective, open-label, 18-month trial of calcium hydroxylapatite (Radiesse) for facial soft-tissue augmentation in patients with human immunodeficiency virus–associated lipoatrophy: one-year durability. *Plastic and Reconstructive Surgery* Sep;**118**(3 Suppl):34S–45S, 2006

Chapter 2

APPROACH TO CHOOSING THE IDEAL FILLER

by

Mary P. Lupo, MD, FAAD

INTRODUCTION

Presently, there is no one ideal filler for all patients, for all indications, and in all situations. It is unlikely that this will ever occur, given the extreme variables in patients and in the goals of aesthetic filler injections. The type of product best for lip injection may not be the best for volumetric cheek filling or for dorsal hand augmentation. The injectable filler best for a young woman with fine skin texture is different than that for an older man with redundant folds or for acne scars. The cost of material, duration of effect, and the social downtime issue all play a role in making the final decision of product choice.

In the end, it is the technical skill of the physician and the familiarity with the product that are the most important factors in the clinical result. This discussion will review the key issues to help the practicing aesthetic physician choose the ideal FDA (Federal Drug Association) approved filler for each patient. Fillers that have not been FDA approved in the United States, autologous fat (an excellent global restorative filler), and silicone (an excellent permanent filler for HIV lipotrophy) will not be discussed here.

CHARACTERISTICS OF THE IDEAL FILLER

The ideal filler is nonallergenic, durable yet reversible, has a natural look and feel after injection, is able to be injected in off-face areas, and is very safe. It should be easy to inject and should cause only little pain, swelling, or bruising. For purposes of being a good business model for a busy practice, it should be prepackaged in sterile vials or syringes, requiring no mixing, and be reasonably priced to be affordable to the patient for many years since return visits ensure a viable practice. If the product does not require skin testing for allergenicity, patients could be injected at the initial consult, which enhances compliance and improves patient conversion, both important for the practice business model. Smaller needle size for patient comfort, yet with ease of flow to prevent hand fatigue for the physician, would be important for an ideal product.

POPULAR FILLER OPTIONS

Presently, in the United States, the FDA is the authoritative body that approves aesthetic fillers as medical devices. Studies that show efficacy and safety must be presented. Devices are not required to have such rigorous testing as drugs, but for more than twenty years, only one type of filler, bovine collagen, was FDA approved. Zyderm I, Zyderm II, and the more cross-linked version, Zyplast revolutionized cosmetic dermatology. They were the "gold standard" for fillers for two decades. Human-derived collagen (Cosmoderm, Cosmoplast) followed in 2003, and then, several hyaluronic acid (HA) products received FDA clearance. These included Restylane, Hylaform, Hylaform Plus, Captique, Juvederm Ultra, Juvederm Ultra Plus, Perlane, Elevess, and Prevelle Silk. Currently, only Restylane, Perlane, Juvederm Ultra and Ultra Plus, and Prevelle Silk are sold in the United States.

Poly-L-lactic acid (PLLA: FDA approved Sculptra), calcium hydroxy apatite (CaHA, Radiesse), polymethyl methacrylate (PMMA, Artefill), and a newly approved porcine cross-linked collagen, Evolence, complete the list of available fillers. Presently, the facial lines and folds are approved for injection of HA, collagen products, CaHA, PLLA and PMMA. CaHA and PLLA are approved for HIV-associated face lipoatrophy. No product is FDA approved for lip augmentation, periorbital injection, glabellar, earlobe augmentation, nor for cosmetic volumetric or cheek enhancement. Since these areas, as well as hands, are not cleared by the FDA and yet are commonly injected, most aesthetic filling is done "off-label" under the discretion of the treating physician.

MAKING THE BEST CHOICE

There are some guidelines that a physician can follow when choosing fillers. The thickness of the patient's skin is one of the first variables that should be considered. Thicker, more robust, structural fillers are

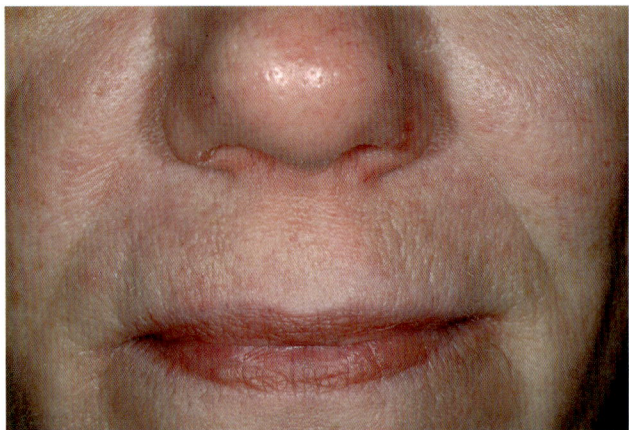

FIG. 2.1.   Sebaceous, thick skin before treatment.

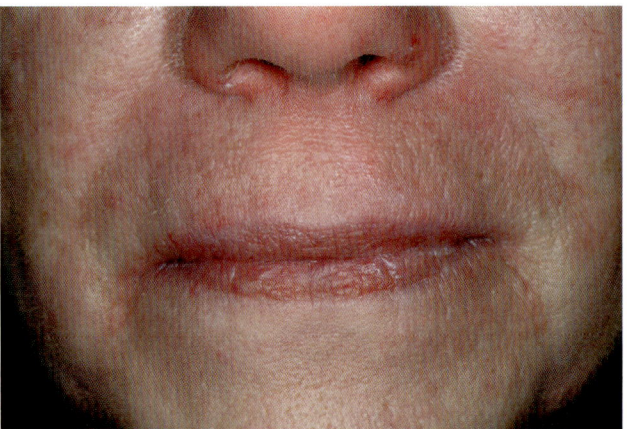

FIG. 2.2.   Sebaceous, thick skin immediately after 2 cc of Perlane.

better for patients with thicker skin, "sebaceous" skin with redundant folds (Figures 2.1 and 2.2). Such products often require less volume to achieve improvement. The concentration of HA and degree of cross-linking of the HA have been found to be important for the characteristics of the final HA product.[1,2] For those products that are particle sized, a larger particle size may translate to greater lift for thicker skin.

The placement and volume of filler injected affect lift in thicker skin. Layering filler at different depths has a beneficial effect for thicker skin as well. In contrast, finer lines or lines that are etched into the skin have fewer complications when injected with

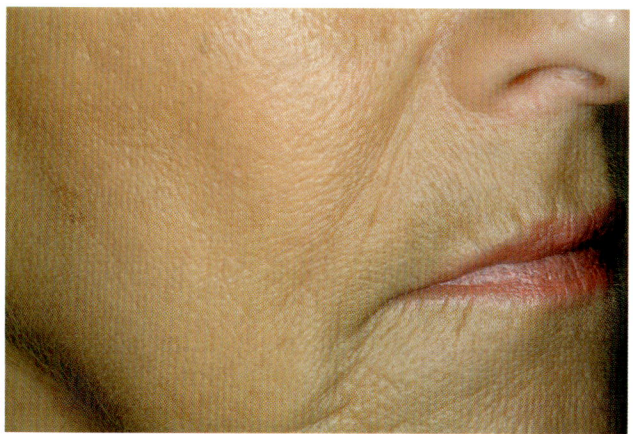

FIG. 2.3.   *Thin delicate skin before treatment.*

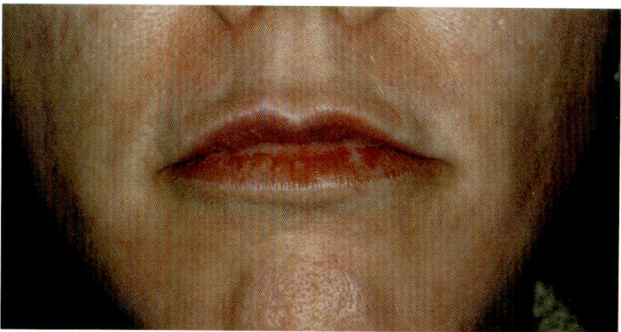

FIG. 2.5.   *Superficial injection of Perlane into finely etched perioral lines lateral to the mouth corners.*

thinner fillers (Figures 2.3 and 2.4). Less viscous fillers are less likely to make the skin heavy and result in out-pouching or lumping, which can occur when heavier products are injected into thin lines (Figures 2.5 and 2.6).

Skin color and ethnic skin variations are important considerations when choosing fillers. Non-Caucasian ethnic groups are one of the fastest growing groups of aesthetic patients. These patients with heavily pigmented skin are at risk for postinflammatory hyperpigmentation (PIH). Some fillers have been specifically tested on heavily pigmented skin and have been found to be safe (Figures 2.7 and 2.8).[3]

Dermatologists who specialize in cosmetic procedures have reported very favorable results with filler use in ethnic skin.[4] Technique changes are important with ethnic skin. Fewer sticks implanted into the skin are singularly important for darker skin because the puncture sites are the most common sites of PIH. More robust fillers, therefore, that give more lift per stick are optimal. In addition, since melanin decreases photoaging, darker skin does not usually require the filling of fine rhytids that respond best to thinner fillers.

Product duration is very important in choosing fillers. More cross-linkage and less free HA concentration have been found to affect duration.[1,2] Particle size has not shown an effect on persistence of correction. Both depth of injection and total volume injected impact duration. Injection of a greater

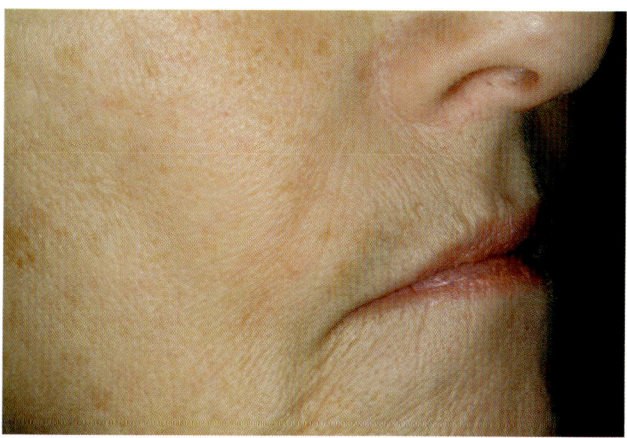

FIG. 2.4.   *Thin delicate skin four months after injecting 0.4 cc of Juvederm Ultra.*

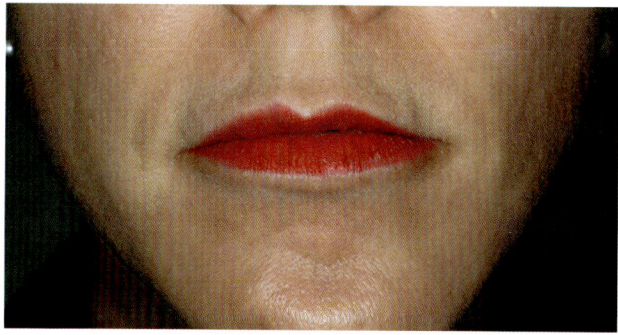

FIG. 2.6.   *Camouflaging the out-pouching with Restylane and Botox.*

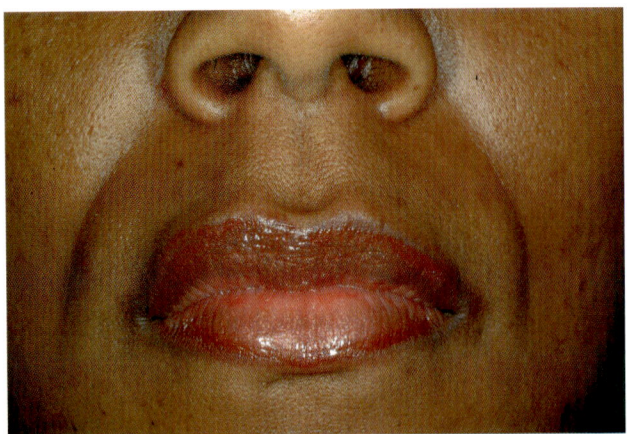

FIG. 2.7. *African American before treatment.*

volume of any type of filler to full correction is associated with longer duration of effect. Variables from patient to patient such as the quality of the skin, patient age, and ongoing exposure to the sun have an effect on duration with the same product. Touch-up injections after full correction require less volume and make filler correction more cost effective over time.[5] In one study comparing the duration of CaHA and HA fillers, less product and longer duration seemed to make the CaHA filler relatively preferred when considering this issue.[6] PMMA, PLLA, and CaHA have a collagen-stimulating effect that results in longer correction duration.

Older skin requires greater volume for correction and has more of an issue with lipoatrophy, so collagen-stimulating fillers are often the better choice. PLLA, approved for folds and wrinkles on July 31, 2009, has found a place in volumetric filling in both older patients and younger patients demonstrating a gaunt appearance from exaggerated facial length as well as from illness or genetically derived low facial fat (Figures 2.9 and 2.10).

The patient's personal preferences are also important considerations. Many patients request "natural" products made of materials found in their bodies. Human collagen and HA, which is identical across species, would likely be their preference. A patient who has been treated with fillers for a number of

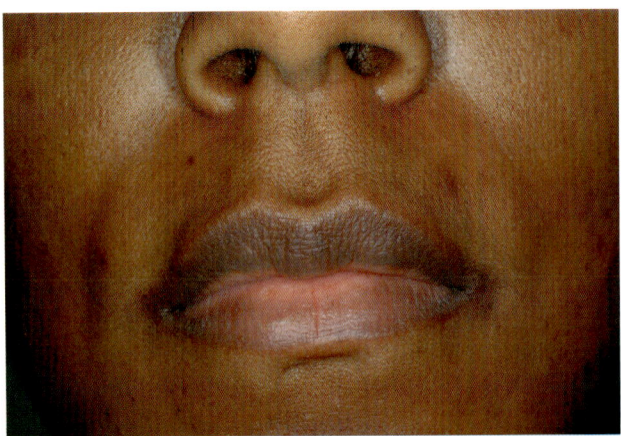

FIG. 2.8. *African American two months after injection of 1.6 cc Juvederm Ultra Plus.*

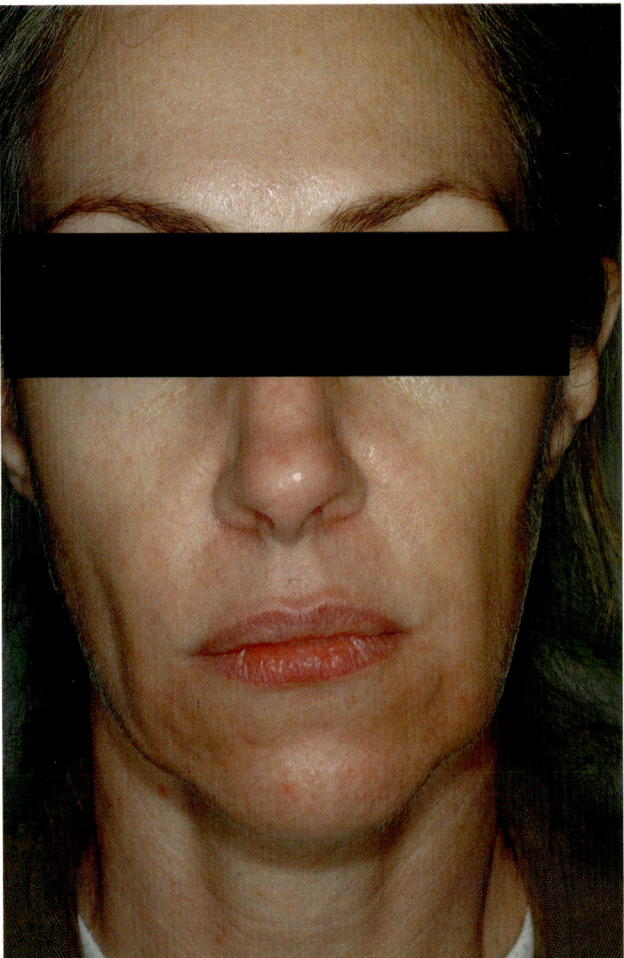

FIG. 2.9. *Gaunt face before treatment.*

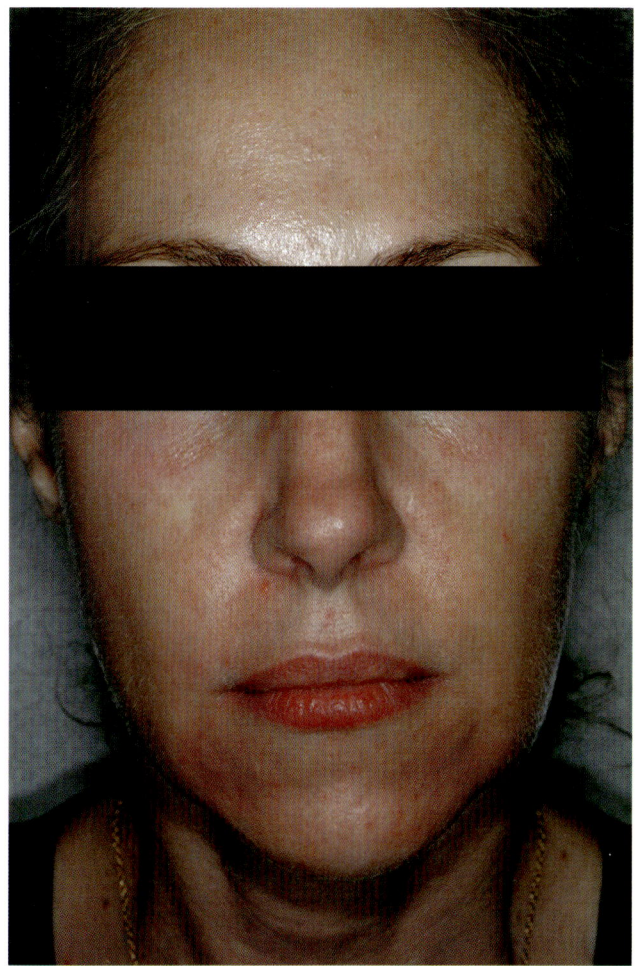

FIG. 2.10.   *Four months after a total of 3 vials Sculptra over three sessions.*

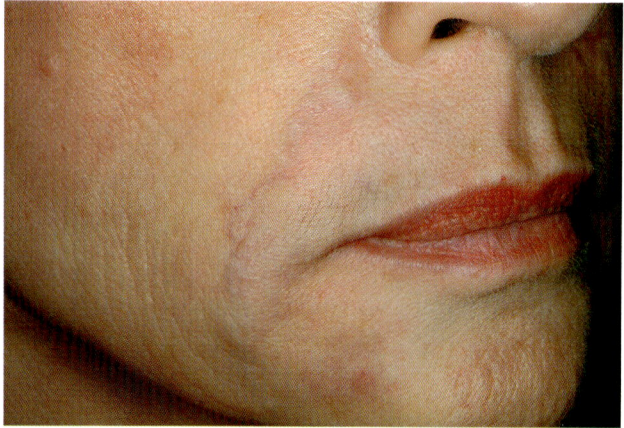

FIG. 2.11.   *Reaction to Restylane six months after injection of 1 cc.*

years may be interested in a permanent filler such as PMMA or silicone, so he or she may discontinue frequent visits for correction. Others may request a treatment that gives results very gradually over time so as to not reveal to others a dramatic change.[7] PLLA is ideal for that situation. Others like the idea of immediate results with the promise of longevity from collagen stimulation and CaHA is the best choice for these patients.

The ability to reverse the correction if the patient is unhappy is the most compelling reason to use HA fillers for hesitant patients (Figures 2.11 and 2.12). Lip injection can result in unhappy patients if the change is too drastic or if it changes the shape of

the lips. For this reason, many patients prefer a shorter duration product first to try the new lips on for size before continuing on to a product known to have greater duration. The problem of immediate swelling or bruising may impact a patient's product preference. Some physicians have reported definite differences in swelling after lip injection when comparing homogenous gel HA versus particle-sized HA filler.[8] In addition, fillers that are in equilibrium with water before injection will result in a "what you see, is what you get" result with no delayed swelling. Tendency for bruising is another consideration when patients require a "no-downtime" treatment, although bruising is more a function of patient

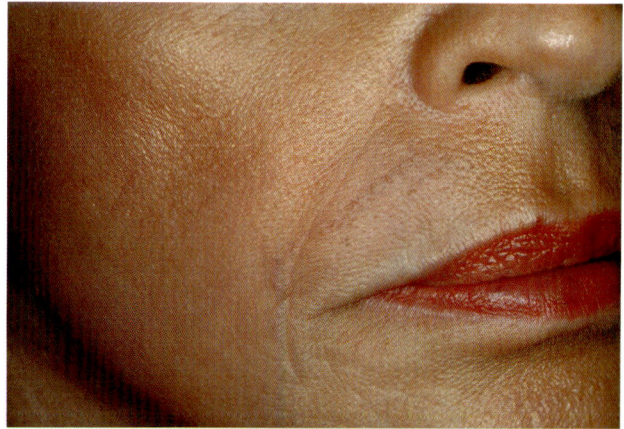

FIG. 2.12.   *Correction of reaction with hyaluronidase one week later.*

propensity, use of aspirin or nonsteroidal medications, fish oil, and vitamin E supplements. Well-designed studies have identified that injection technique, especially slow injection rate, can impact bruising and swelling more than the product choice.[9] Finally, pain and the fear of it are powerful dissuaders. Fillers with added lidocaine are great choices for these patients. Anesthetics are now being added by physicians after manufacturing and there has been no change in the safety effectiveness or duration.[10,11] Fine-gauge needle use is another variable that may affect patient preference. More robust, thicker fillers must be injected with a larger bore needle and may increase the patient's sensation of pain due to the larger bore needle as well as the pressure on tissue from the thicker product.

As mentioned, social downtime considerations must be factored in product choice as human collagen and low-concentration HA are less likely to bruise and swell. This consideration must be weighed with economic issues. Thicker materials and those that stimulate collagen production may be better values in the long run because of superior maintenance of correction.

Within the same patient, there is a need for differing product use. Products such as CaHA, PMMA, and PLLA are poor choices for lip augmentation.

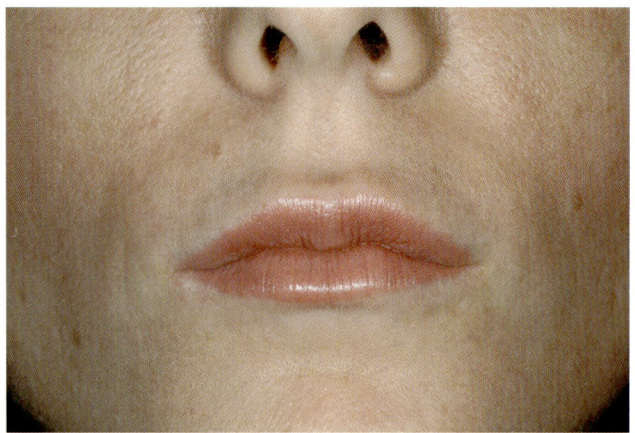

FIG. 2.14.   Nine months after injection of total 0.8 cc Juvederm Ultra Plus into the lips, perioral rhytids, and nasolabial fold in a twenty-eight-year-old female.

Softer and less viscous fillers are better for perioral rhytids and for natural lip augmentation (Figures 2.13 and 2.14).[1,12] The poor vascularity of the glabellar area dictates the need for a less viscous product that can be injected into the upper dermis. Deep dermal injections in this area are considered risky for vascular occlusion and skin necrosis, so large particle-sized HA, CaHA, and PMMA should be avoided. Cheek augmentation does better with a more robust product that can be molded for a natural look. Finally, thicker, collagen-stimulating, structural fillers such as CaHA are good for bound-down acne scars. These types of issues are considered when counseling a patient about filler options.

The author has experience with all these fillers and has formulated opinion to guide the novice injector when it comes to product choice. Some basic fillers with their relative strengths and weaknesses are listed in Table 2.1.

PRECAUTIONS

One final discussion of great importance is the complication issue. Although all fillers have potential complications, the risks with filler use are low. Temporary, self-limiting side effects such as bruising, lumping, swelling, and asymmetry are well known

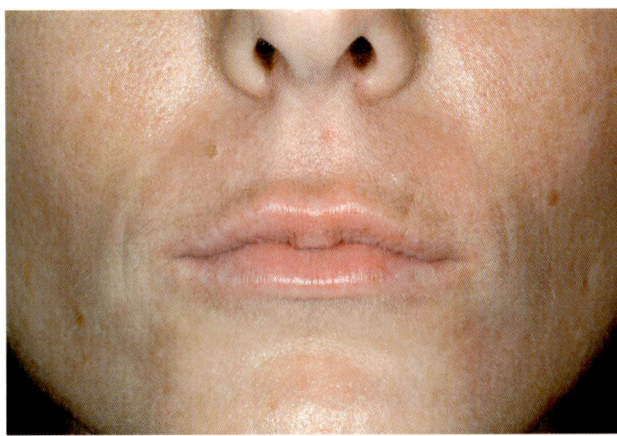

FIG. 2.13.   Before correction.

TABLE 2.1. Product and Relative Strengths/Weaknesses for Use

Product	Strengths	Weaknesses
Bovine collagen (Zyplast, Zyderm)	Long history, little inflammation, bruising, particularly good for fine lines	Requires skin testing, short duration, unavailable 2010
Human-derived collagen (Cosmoderm, Cosmoplast)	Same as bovine collagen, no skin testing, gives structural shape	Short duration, unavailable 2010
Small particle size HA (Restylane)	Consumer popularity, stiffness for shaping, no skin testing, versatile, reversible	More bruising than with collagen, uncross-linked HA needed for extrusion decreases longevity
Larger particle size HA (Perlane)	Good lift for thicker skin, good for cheeks, thick folds, reversible	Larger particle size has not translated into longer duration than smaller particle-sized HA, not for fine lines
Homogenous HA gel 6% cross-linked (Juvederm Ultra Plus)	Smooth flow, good for lips, can be used in fine lines, versatile, reversible	Not good for demarcating lip line, philtral column
Homogenous HA gel 8% cross-linked (Juvederm Ultra Plus)	Good for cheeks, small volume restoration, good duration, reversible	Not good for fine lines, inefficient for large volume restoration
CaHA (Radiesse)	Good for structural lift, efficient for larger volumes giving immediate effect, good duration + collagen stimulation	Not good for lips, superficial injection causes persistent nodules, complications persistent
PLLA (Sculptra)	Good for larger volume restoration, good duration of effect, good for temporal restoration	Cannot use in lips, requires mixing, product pricing an issue, delayed effect, inconsistent effect, if nodules occur, they persist
PMMA (Artefill)	Permanence of effect	Requires skin test, cannot use in lips, side effects permanent
Small particle HA + lidocaine (Prevelle Silk)	Painless, soft product, good for lips, fine lines, little bruising, reversible	Poor duration, not enough lift for deeper folds
Porcine collagen (Evolence)	Little pain, swelling, bruising, good duration, gives structural shape	Not for lips, nodules persist, material sets quickly, so must be massaged and molded quickly. Feels firm in the skin
High concentration HA + lidocaine (Elevess)	Decreased pain	Inflammatory response, sterile abscesses

and indeed possible with any and all choices. Technique, physician inexperience, and patient tendencies are more often the important variables much more than product choice. Potentially catastrophic vascular occlusion and tissue or vision loss have been reported but are exceedingly rare.[13,14] The single issue of significance with filler complication is reversibility. If the material can be quickly removed or dissolved, then any complication can be mitigated more quickly and definitively. In general, the more persistent the product, the longer the duration of complication. Injections that are too superficial in the dermis often persist for months longer than a properly placed product. For these reasons, HA fillers hold the edge, and reversibility is probably the single factor driving their popularity with doctors. Hyaluronidase injections have been proven to work quickly and safely to remove excess or problematic HA

filler.[15,16] Such a cushion is welcome for busy doctors needing to hand-hold patients with complications for many months.

SUMMARY

The practicing aesthetic physician can have complete confidence in currently available FDA-approved fillers. For best results, the treating physician should be well educated in the relative strengths and weaknesses of all products. Proper technique, patient selection, and planning can assure a positive outcome in the aesthetic result.

REFERENCES

1. Falcone SJ, Berg RA. Crosslinked hyaluronic acid dermal fillers: a comparison of rheological properties. *J Biomed Mater Res A.* 2008 Oct; 87(1):264–271.

2. Tezel A, Fredrickson GH. The science of hyaluronic acid. *J Cosmet Laser Ther.* 2008 Mar; 10(1):35–42.

3. Lupo MP, Smith SR, Thomas JA, Murphy DK, Beddingfield FC. Effectiveness of Juvederm Ultra Plus dermal filler in the treatment of severe nasolabial folds. *Plast Reconstr Surg.* 2008; 121:289–297.

4. Burgess CM. Soft tissue augmentation in skin of color: market growth, available fillers, and successful techniques. *J Drugs Dermatol.* 2007; 6(1):51–55.

5. Narins RS, Dayan SH, Brandt FS, Baldwin EK. Persistence and improvement of nasolabial fold correction with nonanimal-stabilized hyaluronic acid 100,000 gel particles/ml filler on two retreatment schedules: results up to 18 month on two retreatment schedules. *Dermatol Surg.* 2008 Jun; 34(Suppl. 1):S2–S8.

6. Moers-Carpi M, Vogt S, Martinez Santos B, Planas J, Rovira Vallve S, Howell DJ. A multicenter, randomized trial comparing calcium hydroxylapatite to two hyaluronic acids for treatment of nasolabial folds. *Dermatol Surg.* 2007; 33(Suppl.2):S144–S151.

7. Lupo MP. Natural look in volume restoration. *J Drugs Dermatol.* 2008; 7(9):833–839.

8. Clark CP. Animal-based hyaluronic acid fillers: scientific and technical considerations. *Plast Reconstr Surg.* 2007; 120(Suppl.):27S–31S.

9. Glogau RG, Kane MAC. Effect of injection techniques on the rate of local adverse events in patients implanted with nonanimal hyaluronic acid gel dermal fillers. *Dermatol Surg.* 2008; 34:S105–S109.

10. Busso M, Voights R. An investigation of changes in physical properties of injectable Ca hydroxylapatite in a carrier gel when mixed with lidocaine and with lidocaine-epinephrine. *Dermatol Surg.* 2008; 34:S16–S24.

11. Lupo MP, Svetman G, Waller W. Comparison of the efficacy and tolerability of non-animal stabilized hyaluronic acid filler with and without lidocaine hydrochloride 2% for the correction of nasolabial folds. Poster presented at: Cosmetic Boot Camp, June 2009. Aspen, Co.

12. Smith KC. Practical use of Juvederm: early experience. *Plast Reconstr Surg.* 2007; 120(Suppl.):67S–73S.

13. Lowe NJ, Maxwell CA, Patnaik R. Adverse reactions to dermal fillers. *Dermatol Surg.* 2005; 31:1616–1625.

14. Lemperle G, Rullan PP, Gauthier-Hazan N. Avoiding and treating dermal filler complications. *Plast Reconstr Surg.* 2006; 118(3 Suppl.):92S–107S.

15. Hirsch RJ, Lupo MP, Cohen JL, Duffy D. Delayed presentation of impending necrosis following soft tissue augmentation with hyaluronic acid and successful management with hyaluronidase. *J Drugs Dermatol.* 2007; 6:325–328.

16. Brody HJ. Use of hyaluronidase in the treatment of granulomatous hyaluronic acid reactions or unwanted hyaluronic acid misplacement. *Dermatol Surg.* 2005; 31:893–897.

Chapter 3

PATIENT SELECTION, COUNSELING, AND INFORMED CONSENT

by

Sumit Bapna, MD and Corey S. Maas, MD

INTRODUCTION

Dermal fillers have been available for more than 100 years, originally as injectable fat and more recently as biocompatible soft tissue fillers. The use of fillers has continued to increase in cosmetic surgery practices with the greater demands from patients for aesthetic improvement without surgery.[1–6] This increase is secondary to not only the growing indications and availability of dermal fillers but also the desire for rejuvenation from a wider patient population among varying age groups and ethnicities.[6] Currently available dermal fillers include porcine, bovine, and human collagens, hyaluronic acid (HA) preparations of animal or biosynthetic origin, poly-L-lactic acid products, polymethacrylate, and calcium hydroxyapatite. The use of soft tissue fillers is an attractive office procedure for providers because of the associated ease, cost, and minimal discomfort involved in treatment. Although the use of injectable soft tissue fillers is relatively safe, it is important to select patients carefully and counsel them appropriately to avoid complications. The process of informed consent is a crucial component of the relationship that must develop between the provider and the patient to minimize the already rare occurrence of legal complications.[6]

PATIENT SELECTION

The media and manufacturer marketing has instilled views and expectations of complete rejuvenation of facial aging in patients by the use of fillers. Patient selection is important to have satisfied patients and reduce undesired outcomes. A thorough review of the history is the first step in this process. Excessive bleeding, bruising, or abnormal scar formation should be documented, and the patient should be aware that this may occur as a result of dermal filler injection. History of anaphylactoid reactions, lidocaine hypersensitivity, and previous bovine collagen hypersensitivity should also be elicited before considering bovine collagen for tissue augmentation. As part of the patient's history, it is important to know that the patient has realistic expectations. Patients should also be psychologically stable without conditions such as body dysmorphic disorder, depression, or obsessive-compulsive disorder.[6] The patient's goals should be discussed so that we, the providers, can direct them to reasonable and appropriate alternatives if fillers are not felt to be appropriate for their expected results.

Frequently, patients obtain information from multiple sources, including newspaper, television, and other media controlled by the manufacturer. The FDA can only control what the manufacturer states, not what the journalists write in marketing stories.[4] It is imperative that the physician/provider do not succumb to patient demands for unapproved products and unreachable goals.

COUNSELING

In addition to good patient selection, pretreatment counseling can help minimize complications. It is very important that the physician and the patient discuss the desired outcome and agree upon realistic expectations. The provider needs to remain the expert in discussing the expected results and the product that would best achieve the goals of the patient. Otherwise, the physician/provider may be forced to accept liability when he/she predictably fails to deliver his or her goals. For example, if a patient is new and hesitant, a more temporary therapy can be suggested initially. In this manner, less time elapses until resolution of the unsatisfying result.[6]

A large portion of patient counseling involves discussing the possible complications associated with treatment. In regard to soft tissue fillers, two types of complications should be discussed: The acute reactions can include edema, pain, erythema, bleeding, ecchymosis, and nodularity. Delayed and more significant reactions include migration of implant material, incorrect injection site, inadequate/excessive injection of material, allergic reaction to implant material, inflammatory/granulomatous/autoimmune reactions, dyspigmentation, infectious complications, scarring, acne, and/or tissue infarction.[1–7] The relative infrequency of these complications should be

communicated, but the consequences of complications should not be minimized.

Another aspect of patient counseling is documenting and making patients aware of facial asymmetry. Photodocumentation, before and after treatment, can assist in this capacity as well as in explaining expected results and making expectations reasonable and realistic.[6]

INFORMED CONSENT

Obtaining informed consent is a crucial component in minimizing legal complications. Informed consent is a process by which patients learn about their options and choices, the procedure, the product, inherent risks, complications, and required medication-related issues. The two national standards are (1) what a reasonable patient needs to know to make an informed decision about his or her care and (2) what a reasonable doctor needs to tell the patient to make an informed decision about his or her care.[4] The physician should be very comfortable using the offered fillers and handling potential complications as well as must know how to avoid them so that patients are well informed and can appropriately participate in the consent.

Consent forms can be standardized for a particular practice as the risks for dermal fillers are common to most products. Additional text can be added for more permanent fillers. Also since results should not be guaranteed verbally, consent forms should reflect this as well.

It is important to provide patients with comprehensive information about soft tissue fillers as a component of the informed consent process. This should consist of both verbal discussion and written information to cater to different learning styles. The verbal discussion is conducted throughout the pretreatment interview. The details of the risks, benefits, alternatives, and potential complications can be discussed when the paper form, signifying informed consent, is signed.

However, discussion of risks should not be exclusive to the immediate pretreatment period, as patients should have sufficient time to consider the information. Prior studies have shown that only 35–50 percent of what is said to the patient is retained. Written information, in the form of copies of consents and product brochures, can increase the percentage of information retained by patients.[4,8] Providing the written consent to the patients before the actual physician discussion is practical in that it can save time for the physician and also expedite care because patients can have time to formulate questions they may have after reading the consent form (Figure 3.1).

It should be stressed to the prospective patient that complications do occur. It is important to be honest to patients. The common complications mentioned earlier should be discussed verbally, although discussion of the uncommon complications can be reserved for the written consent form. This should increase the number of highly pleased and satisfied patients and decrease legal complications.

CONCLUSION

The use of fillers for soft tissue augmentation will probably continue to increase as more products with different compositions and characteristics are introduced and approved for use and as the aging population continues to search for minimally invasive rejuvenating procedures. It is important for physicians who provide treatment with fillers to understand the advantages and disadvantages of one filler over another and appreciate the limitations of their use so that patients continue to stay well informed. With this thorough understanding, both the patient and the physician can be active in the process of informed consent. When physicians and patients take informed consent seriously, the patient–physician relationship becomes a true partnership with shared decision-making authority and responsibility

Consent for Hyaluronic Acid

Restylane or Juvederm or Perlane

I _____, elect to have the above procedure performed and I understand that this procedure is for cosmetic purposes only, not for health reasons. The nature of the above procedure has been explained to me. I am advised that although good results are expected, complications cannot be anticipated, therefore no guarantee can be either expressed or implied as to the final results of the above procedure.

Juvederm, Restylane and Perlane injectable gels are colorless hyaluronic acid gels that are injected into facial tissue to smooth wrinkles and folds, especially around the nose and mouth. Hyaluronic acid is a naturally occurring sugar found in the human body. The role of hyaluronic acid in the skin is to deliver nutrients, hydrate the skin by holding in water, and to act as a cushioning agent. Juvederm, Restylane and Perlane injectable gels are injected into areas of facial tissue where moderate to severe facial wrinkles and folds occur. It temporarily adds volumes to the skin and may give the appearance of a smoother surface. Most patients need one treatment to achieve optimal wrinkle smoothing, and the results last about six months.

Risks of the above procedure are:

- Bruising or bleeding at the injection site
- Possible infection
- Swelling
- Vascular occlusion
- Localized necrosis and/or sloughing of tissue
- Vision loss

I request the above procedure, appreciating and accepting the permanency of the procedure, as well as the complications and consequences of the procedure. I understand that some temporary superficial bruising occurs in some patients and may require make up to conceal any temporary superficial bruising. The RN and/or MD have explained to me the most likely complication or problems that may occur with this procedure and during the healing period, and I understand them. I have had sufficient opportunity to discuss my condition and treatment with the RN and/or MD, and all questions have been answered to my satisfaction. I am also aware that I may discuss my procedure with another RN and/or MD if I elect to do so. I believe that I have adequate knowledge upon which to base an informed consent to the purposed procedure.

Patient Signature_____

Date_____

Witness_____

FIG. 3.1. *Sample informed consent form.*

for outcomes.[9] The use of informed consent for dermal fillers may not be the standard of care but it would be foolish not to obtain it.

REFERENCES

1. Narins RS, Brandt FS, Lorenc ZP, Maas CS, Monheit GD, Smith SR. Twelve-month persistency of a novel ribose-cross-linked collagen dermal filler. *Dermatologic Surgery.* 2008; **34**:S31–S39.

2. Narins RS, Brandt FS, Lorenc ZP, Maas CS, Monheit GD, Smith SR, McIntyre S. A randomized multicenter study of the safety and efficacy of Dermicol-P35 and non-animal-stabilized hyaluronic acid gel for the correction of nasolabial folds. *Dermatologic Surgery.* 2007; **33**:S213–S221.

3. Eppley BL, Dadvand B. Injectable soft-tissue fillers: clinical overview. *Plastic and Reconstructive Surgery.* 2006; **118**:98e–106e.

4. Reisman NR. Ethics, legal issues, and consent for fillers. *Clinics in Plastic Surgery.* 2006; **33**:505–510.

5. Ali MJ, Ende K, Maas CS. Perioral rejuvenation and lip augmentation. *Facial Plastic Surgery Clinics of North America.* 2006; **15**:491–500.

6. Engelman DE, Bloom B, Goldberg DJ. Dermal fillers: complications and informed consent. *Journal of Cosmetic and Laser Therapy.* 2005; **7**:29–32.

7. Maas CS. Botulinum neurotoxins and injectable fillers: minimally invasive management of the aging upper face. *Facial Plastic Surgery Clinics of North America.* 2006; **14**:241–245.

8. Makdessian AS, Ellis DA, Irish JC. Informed consent in facial plastic surgery; effectiveness of a simple educational intervention. *Archives of Facial Plastic Surgery.* 2004; **6**:26–30.

9. Paterick TJ, Carson GV, Allen MC, Paterick TE. Medical informed consent: general considerations for physicians. *Mayo Clinic Proceedings.* 2008; **83**:313–319.

Chapter 4

HYALURONIC ACID SKIN DERIVATIVES

by

Robert Anolik, MD and Ellen Gendler, MD

EMERGENCE OF HYALURONIC ACIDS

As we age, the underlying connective tissue responsible for the skin's youthful elasticity and fullness degenerates. This degeneration is exacerbated by several factors, especially sun exposure and repeated use of underlying muscles. These factors are particularly evident in facial skin. Crow's feet, laugh lines, and smile lines are among the most common cosmetic complaints. Consequently, a fervent desire exists to employ effective and safe cosmetic treatments to bolster the underlying tissue and mitigate these changes. Injectable fillers have proven to be an effective method of achieving this goal.

The first FDA-approved cosmetic filler that generated substantial enthusiasm was collagen. These products, though effective, had substantial drawbacks, including limited longevity and concerns for allergic reaction. The demand for a filler that not only bypassed the need for allergy testing but also offered greater longevity inspired the development of additional fillers, notably hyaluronic acid agents. In December 2003, Restylane became the first FDA approved hyaluronic acid product offered in the United States, and several others have since followed or are pending approval. Aside from longevity and low allergenicity, these newer fillers offer other advantages. Particularly valuable are their inherent ability to bind large amounts of water to further bolster rhytids and cosmetic effect.

EXAMPLES OF HYALURONIC ACIDS

Clinicians use several varieties of hyaluronic acids, including FDA-approved agents such as Restylane, Perlane, Juvederm, Hylaform, Hylaform Plus, Captique, Elevess, and Prevelle Silk. Other hyaluronic acid products, many of which are already used internationally, are expected to be approved by the FDA in the near future.

Restylane, FDA approved in December 2003, is a non–animal stabilized hyaluronic acid (NASHA) produced from streptococcal bacterial fermentation.[1] The acids are cross-linked with 1,4-butanediol diglycidal ether (BDDE). The Restylane family maintains a hyaluronic acid concentration of 20 mg/ml and includes Restylane, Perlane, Restylane Fine Lines, and Restylane SubQ. Perlane achieved FDA approval in May 2007, whereas Restylane Fine Lines and Restylane SubQ have not been approved as of the writing of this text. Perlane comprises relatively larger particle sizes intended for deeper tissue placement, whereas Restylane Fine Lines comprises smaller particles intended for more superficial placement. Restylane SubQ is being designed as a replacement for autologous fat (Figures 4.9 and 4.10).

Juvederm, FDA approved in June 2006, also consists of hyaluronic acid derived from NASHA produced from streptococcal bacterial fermentation. Like Restylane, these acids are cross-linked with BDDE. Unlike other hyaluronic acids, however, Juvederm consists of more homogenous particles that allegedly decrease degradation and increase longevity.[2] This assertion, however, remains unproven.[2] Juvederm maintains a hyaluronic acid concentration of 24 mg/ml and is available in different formulations, including Juvederm Ultra and Juvederm Ultra Plus, which are intended for different levels of dermal placement (Figures 4.1–4.8).

Hylaform, FDA approved in April 2004, comprises hyaluronic acid derived from the dermis of rooster combs. The purified hyaluronic acid is cross-linked with divinyl sulfone (DVS). The Hylaform family maintains a hyaluronic acid concentration of 5.5 mg/ml and includes Hylaform, Hylaform Plus, and Hylaform Fineline. Hylaform Plus achieved FDA approval in October 2004, and, like Perlane, it comprises relatively larger particle sizes that are intended for deeper tissue placement. Hylaform Fineline, like Restylane Fine Lines, comprises relatively smaller particle sizes and is intended for more superficial placement. Hylaform Fineline has not been approved by the FDA as of the writing of this text.

Captique, FDA approved in December 2004, is another NASHA produced from streptococcal bacterial fermentation. The acids are cross-linked with DVS and maintain a hyaluronic acid concentration of 5.5 mg/ml. Although derived from a different source, Captique and Hylaform have equivalent concentrations, degrees of cross-linking, cross-linking agents, and gel particle size.

Elevess, FDA approved in July 2007, consists of NASHA produced from streptococcal bacterial fermentation and maintains a hyaluronic acid concentration of 28 mg/ml. Elevess distinguishes itself from its predecessors most notably by containing 0.3 percent lidocaine as a component of the treatment syringe. Its cross-linker, *p*-phenylene bisethyl carbodiimide (BCDI) is also distinctive. The lidocaine is intended to diminish injection site pain.

Prevelle Silk, FDA approved in March 2008, is the most recent NASHA approved by the FDA. The acids are cross-linked with DVS and maintain a hyaluronic acid concentration of 5.5 mg/ml. Like Elevess, Prevelle Silk contains lidocaine.

Additional hyaluronic acid fillers that have not been approved by the FDA at the time of writing this text but are in use outside of the United States include Teosyal, Esthelis, Puragen, Puragen Plus (contains lidocaine), Dermalive, and Dermadeep. These agents are also NASHA products, though Dermalive and Dermadeep have acrylic hydrogel incorporated.

All of the agents discussed offer immediate cosmetic effects that may last several months at minimum. Newer agents are targeting longer duration, with some claiming the combination product of Dermalive and Dermadeep lasts for several years.[3]

WHAT ARE HYALURONIC ACIDS?

Hyaluronic acid is a glycosaminoglycan, a form of polysaccharide, consisting of repeating D-glucuronic acid and D-*N*-acetylglucosamine disaccharide units.[4]

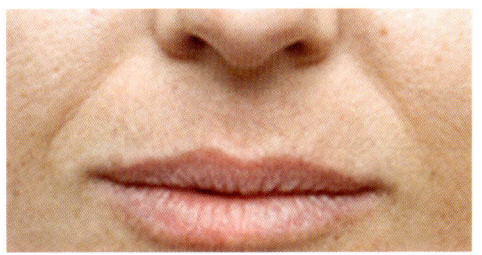

FIG. 4.1. Before 1 cc of Juvederm Ultra.

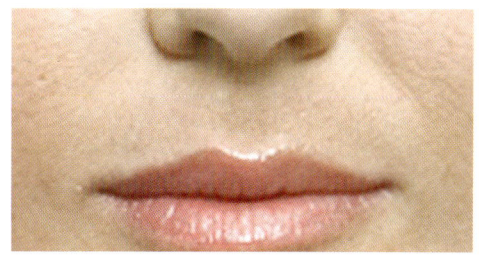

FIG. 4.2. After 1 cc of Juvederm Ultra.

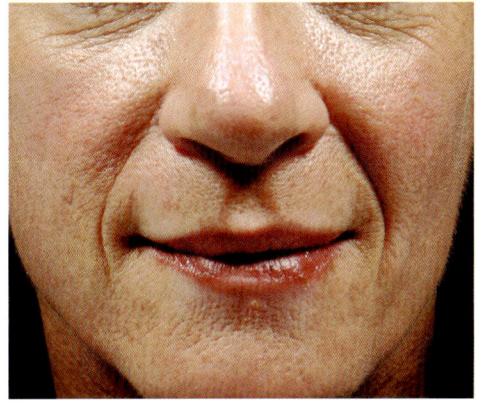

FIG. 4.3. Before 2 cc of Juvederm Ultra.

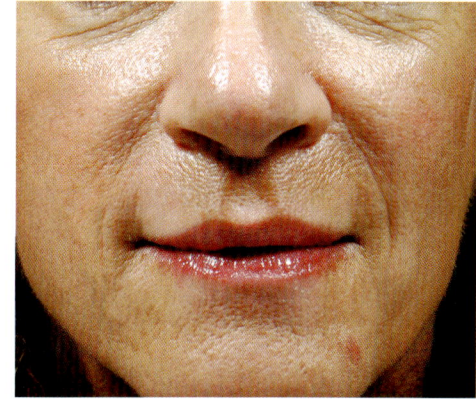

FIG. 4.4. After 2 cc of Juvederm Ultra.

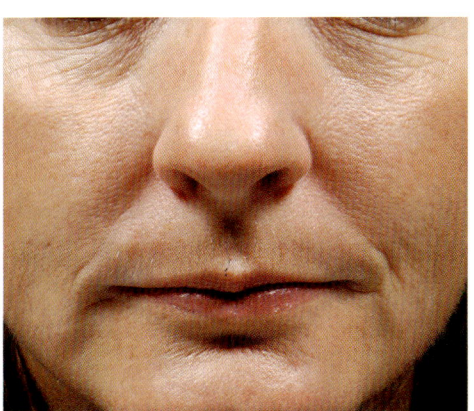

FIG. 4.5. Before 1 cc of Juvederm Ultra Plus.

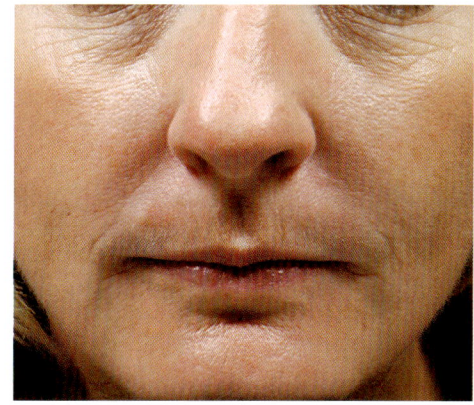

FIG. 4.6. After 1 cc of Juvederm Ultra Plus.

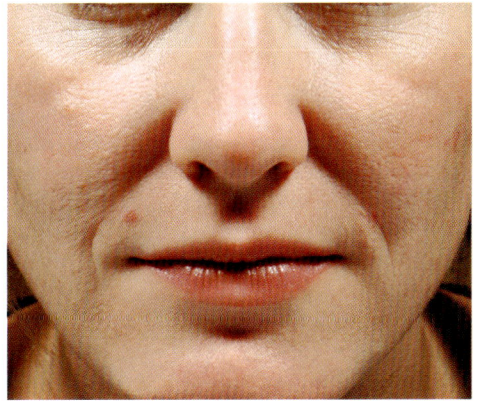

FIG. 4.7. Before 2 cc of Juvederm Ultra Plus.

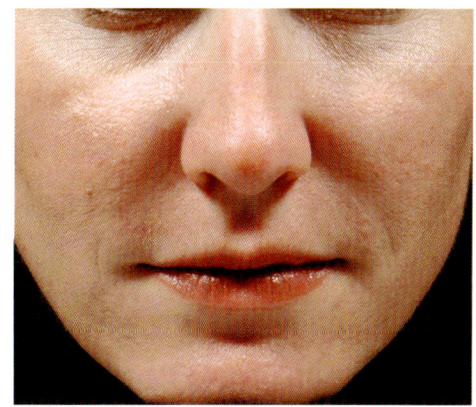

FIG. 4.8. After 2 cc of Juvederm Ultra Plus.

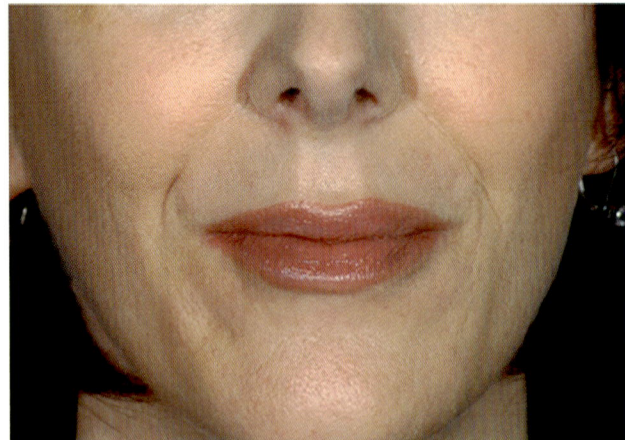

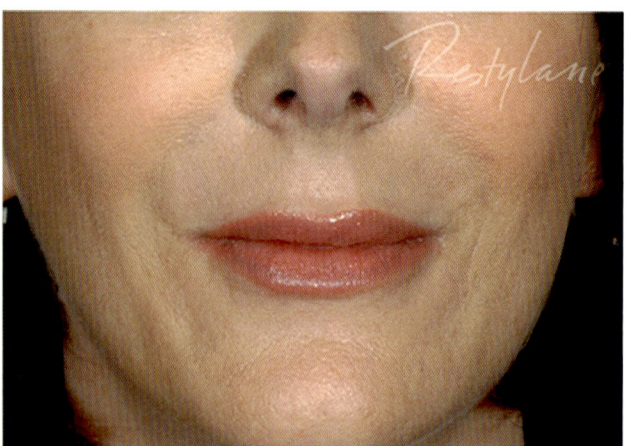

Before treatment
of nasolabial folds

After two *Restylane*® 1 mL syringes
Individual results may vary

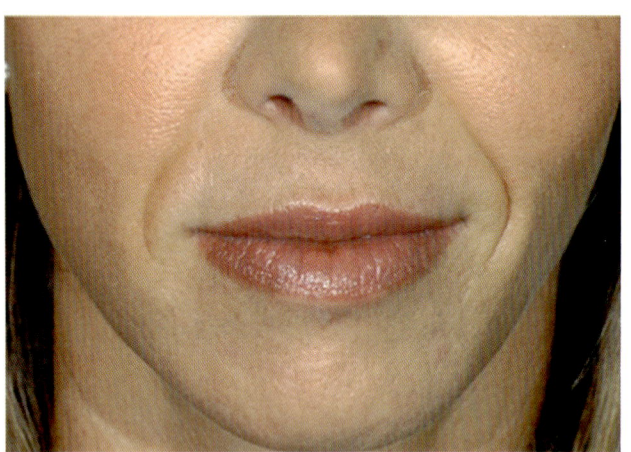

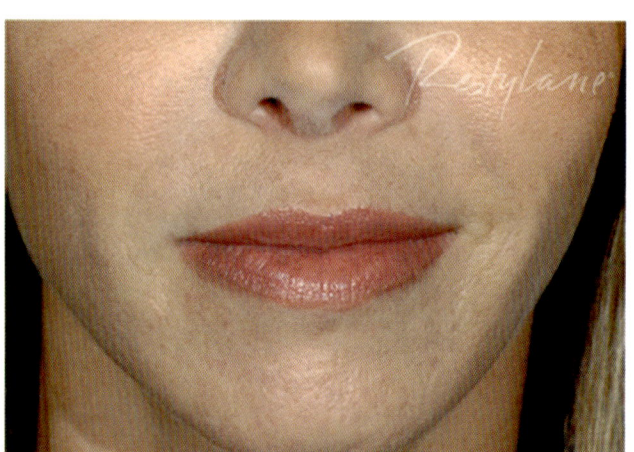

Before treatment
of nasolabial folds

After three *Restylane*® 1 mL syringes
Individual results may vary

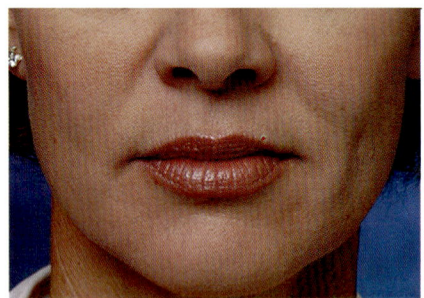

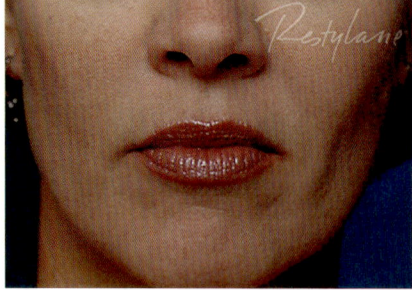

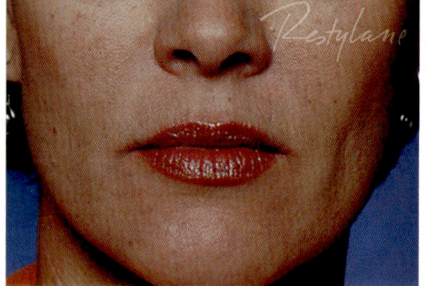

Before treatment
of nasolabial folds

After one *Restylane*® 1 mL syringe
Individual results may vary

After two *Restylane*® 1 mL syringes
Individual results may vary

FIG. 4.9.   Before and after Restylane use (Contact Sheet, Restylane).

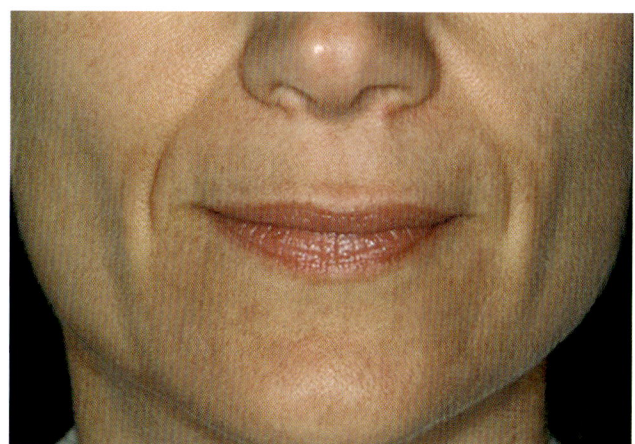

Before treatment
of nasolabial folds

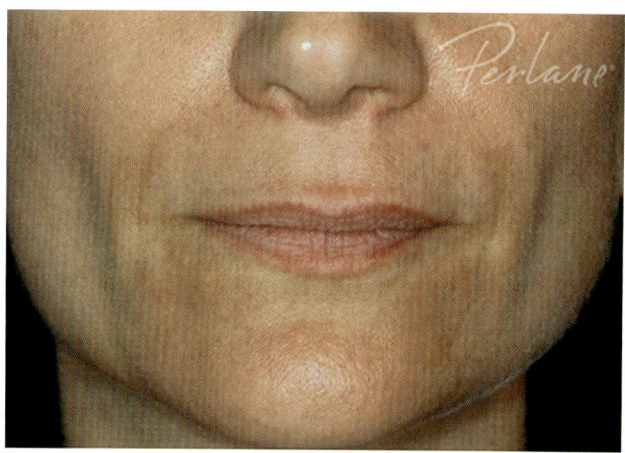

After two *Perlane*® 1 mL syringes
Individual results may vary

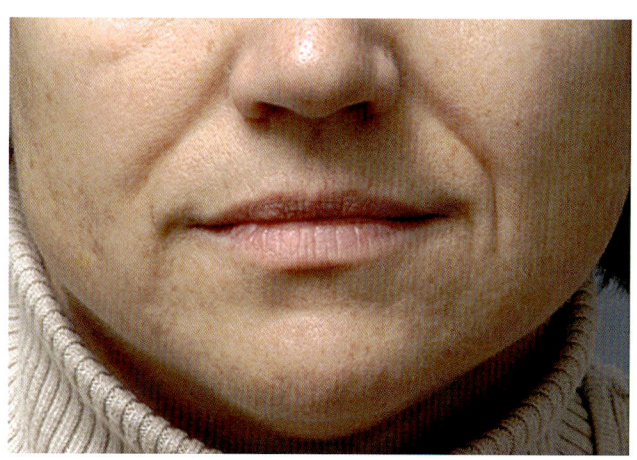

Before treatment
of nasolabial folds

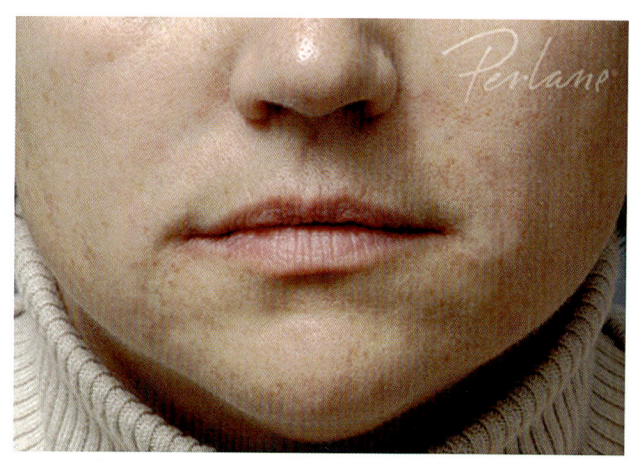

After 2.5 *Perlane*® 1 mL syringes
Individual results may vary

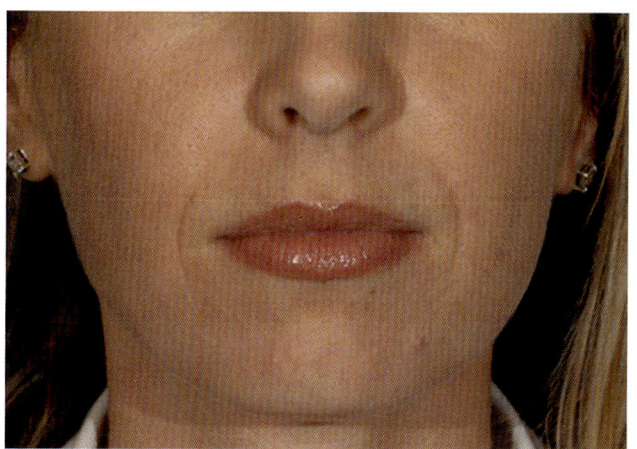

Before treatment
of nasolabial folds

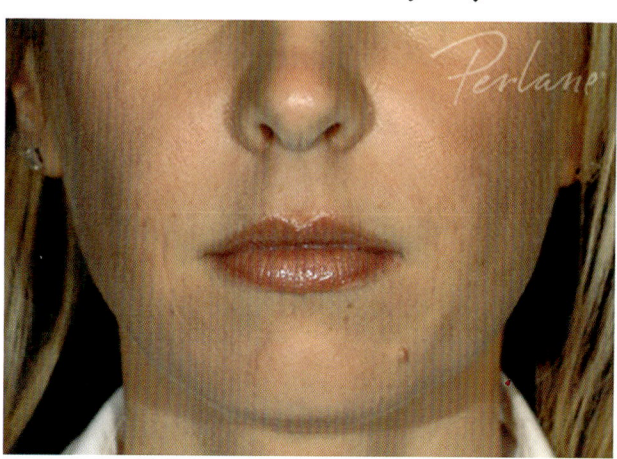

After four *Perlane*® 1 mL syringes
Individual results may vary

FIG. 4.10.   Before and after Perlane use (Contact Sheet, Perlane).

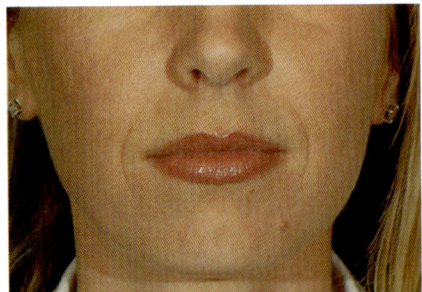
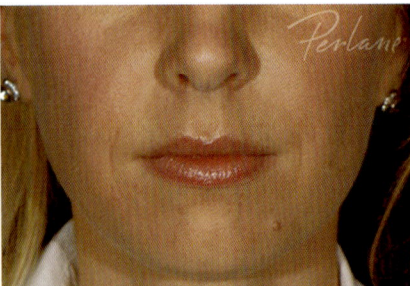
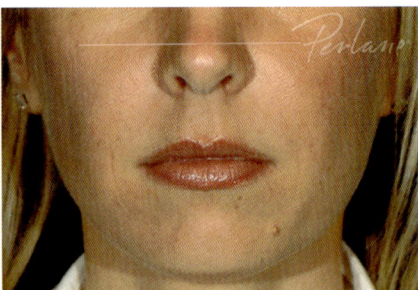

Before treatment
of nasolabial folds

After two *Perlane*® 1 mL syringes
Individual results may vary

After four *Perlane*® 1 mL syringes
Individual results may vary

FIG. 4.10.   (cont.)

The disaccharide unit is often viewed as a monomer that, when bound by beta-1,4 glycosidic bonds, produces a hyaluronic acid polymer.[4] These repeating monomer units can extend up to and beyond 25,000 units, creating molecules with molecular weights greater than 10 MDa.[4]

Endogenous hyaluronic acid is one of the most prevalent glycosaminoglycans in the human dermis and is not species or organ specific.[5,6] In fact, it has been found with an identical structure throughout species as variable as *Pseudomonas*, *Ascaris*, rabbit, and human.[7] Animal-based and bacterial-based hyaluronic acids, both of which are commercially available, differ primarily by length.[4] Animal-based acids tend to have longer polymer chains.

Hyaluronic acid maintains the capacity to bind large quantities of water, which stems from its hydrophilicity. Each disaccharide monomer carries four hydroxyl (–OH) groups and a –COO-Na+ salt group.[4] In an aqueous environment, these hydroxyl groups form hydrogen bonding with water, and the salt group dissociates with a favorable release of energy.[4]

HOW THE HYALURONIC ACID DERMAL FILLERS DIFFER IN CHARACTER

Although the fundamental monomer units of hyaluronic acids are the same, several traits distinguish the range of hyaluronic acid products from one another. Notable variations include the polymer chain length, the degree and type of molecular cross-linking, the gel hardness, the particle size, the required extrusion force, and the extent of hydration.

The polymer chain length and molecular cross-linking traits of a given product are figuratively and literally intertwined. The chain length directly influences hyaluronic acid viscosity and, consequently, longevity by simple entanglement.[7] Entanglement alone, however, builds only a rudimentary network scaffold. Molecular cross-linking of hyaluronic acid polymers stabilizes the network, like the mortar between bricks. When free hyaluronic acid polymer powder is simply mixed into a water solution, a viscous white fluid is produced.[4] If injected into the skin in this free form, the viscous fluid disperses within a few days secondary to water dilution, endogenous hyaluronidase, and free radicals.[4] Clearance would ultimately be achieved by the liver's conversion of the dispersed acid into water and carbon dioxide.[6]

Manufacturers prevent the rapid clearance of the filler by intermixing cross-linkers into the hyaluronic acid preparation. Most commonly, the cross-linkers are BDDE, as found in Restylane and Juvederm, and DVS, as found in Hylaform and Captique. Cross-linkers fortify the hyaluronic acid polymer network by binding the various hydroxyl sites, though the degree of cross-linking varies among different filler products.[1]

Although a higher degree of cross-linking increases stability and longevity, too great a degree has disadvantages. Too high levels of cross-linking can disturb the hydrophilicity and, therefore, the cosmetically desired lifting capacity by diminishing water volume.[4] Furthermore, its deviation from naturally occurring hyaluronic acids could theoretically prompt an immune reaction, thereby producing undesirable granules or abscesses.[4] Additionally, too high degrees of cross-linking can hinder conformation into the targeted cosmetic deficiency as well as increase the required extrusion force from medical devices.[4]

Therefore, manufacturers attempt to achieve a balance between cross-linked and uncross-linked components. Uncross-linked components mitigate the challenges listed in the previous paragraph. Moreover, the uncross-linked components literally act as a lubricant in the filler administration. This lubricating feature of uncross-linked hyaluronic acid has been well documented and is advantageous in other hyaluronic acid applications, such as intra-articular joint injections for osteoarthritis.[7] Taken together, manufacturers must consider the low and high thresholds of cross-linking in their end products.

Gel hardness also plays a role in the characteristics of hyaluronic acid fillers. Polymer scientists describe a variable G', the elastic or storage modulus, to quantify gel hardness. Hardness, or G', represents the force required to hold a given deformation in a gel product.[4] A greater G' implies a harder gel and, clinically, a greater extrusion force in product administration.

Particle size represents another differentiating characteristic among hyaluronic acid products and is dependent on proprietary manufacturing methods.

When initially produced by the manufacturer, gel blocks of hyaluronic acid are formed that are too large for administration. One method of breaking down the gel into usable material is a sieve method, which generally produces a granular end product with particles of an average size. Another method for converting the gel to a usable product is a homogenization process, which produces a less granular product consisting of particles spanning a spectrum of sizes.[4] This method may lower the G' value and ease the extrusion process. Whatever method is employed to break down the initial gel block, the clinician should have an appreciation for a given product's ultimate particle size. The sizes are designed for different dermal depths and affect clinical outcome. For example, the family of Restylane products includes Perlane, Restylane, and Restylane Fine Lines. These three products share an identical hyaluronic acid concentration of 20 mg/ml and chemical composition, though they comprise different particle sizes. Perlane, Restylane, and Restylane Fine Lines contain 10,000, 100,000, and 200,000 particles per milliliter, respectively. Hylaform, Juvederm, and other hyaluronic acid fillers are manufactured with similar models of product families. The greater the size, the more viscous is the filler. Larger particle products may restore greater volume for deep furrows when injected into the deep dermis, but their low viscosity could result in unwanted nodules and irregularities if injected too superficially. Similarly, smaller particle products may allow for correction of superficial lines with less chance of irregularity formation when injected into the superficial dermis but would offer inconsequential results if injected too deeply.

Many traits of hyaluronic acids overlap and influence each other, just as several of the traits already discussed affect the extrusion force character of the syringe-based hyaluronic acid filler products. When the syringe plunger is pressed at a steady rate, the force increases linearly with displacement.[4] With

TABLE 4.1. Summary of FDA-Approved Hyaluronic Acid Fillers

Product	FDA Approval	Cross-Linker	Derivation	Hyaluronic Acid Concentration (mg/ml)	Intermixed Lidocaine	Injection Depth
Restylane	Dec 03	BDDE	NASHA	20	No	Mid-dermis
Perlane	Mar 07	BDDE	NASHA	20	No	Deep dermis
Hylaform	Apr 04	DVS	Avian	5.5	No	Mid-dermis
Hylaform Plus	Oct 04	DVS	Avian	5.5	No	Deep dermis
Captique	Dec 04	DVS	NASHA	5.5	No	Mid-dermis
Juvederm	Jun 06	BDDE	NASHA	24	No	Juvederm Ultra – mid-dermis; Juvederm Ultra Plus – deep dermis
Elevess	Jul 07	BCDI	NASHA	28	Yes	Mid-dermis
Prevelle Silk	Mar 08	DVS	NASHA	5.5	Yes	Mid-dermis

BDDE = 1,4-butanediol diglycidal ether; DVS = divinyl sulfone; BCDI = p-phenylene bisethyl carbodiimide; NASHA = nonanimal stabilized hyaluronic acid.

greater forces, a yield point is achieved at which time the displacement force falls slightly and continuous flow is nearly constant.[4] Therefore, regardless of the extrusion force requirements of a given product, the force-to-displacement curve reveals that more effort is required to start and stop injection as compared to continuous administration.[4]

Finally, the extent of hyaluronic acid hydration influences its character. As mentioned earlier, one of the greatest advantages of hyaluronic acids is their ability to bind large quantities of water. In fact, 1 g of lightly cross-linked hyaluronic acid can bind up to 3 l of water.[4] This advantageous characteristic offers several benefits. One benefit is the product's ability to build substantial volume by accumulation of surrounding water. A less obvious but particularly valuable benefit is the hyaluronic acid filler's ability to maintain similarly high levels of water, even as it slowly degrades. This filler's maintenance of volume until near total degradation is known as isovolemic degradation.[8] Therefore, unlike other biodegradable implants, the hyaluronic acid filler effect does not wane linearly over time and can be reinforced with additional treatments as needed before notable loss of effect.

The great ability to bind water warrants appreciation of each product's hydration state before administration. One could imagine the unpredictable effects of a filler that is not near its expected equilibrium concentration of acid-to-water once that filler is in the skin. In other words, if too high a concentration of acid-to-water were administered into the skin, a too dramatic and possibly unpredictable volumizing effect could result. The opposite would be true for too low a concentration. In general, hyaluronic acid filler products are produced minimally below equilibrium concentration allowing for control and predictable volume gain.

HOW HYALURONIC ACIDS ARE USED

Several guidelines exist for the administration of hyaluronic acid fillers and each clinician may develop variations on these themes.

Appropriate positioning of the clinician and patient will influence the cosmetic outcome. Stability and comfort of both are essential for optimal results. Additionally, many believe real-time assessment of the patient's wrinkles and furrows is valuable to visualizing targeted areas. Therefore, having the patient seated in the upright position with the clinician facing the patient should permit mutual comfort and optimally elucidate gravity and light effects on the patient's targeted areas. Having a headrest or other form of support can diminish unintended movements.

The patient's face should be without makeup to limit risks of foreign body reactions and should also be antiseptically cleaned with products such as alcohol to prevent infection. Gloves should be changed immediately if intraoral manipulation is required to limit any bacterial contamination of the injection sites.[2] If medically able, patients should avoid aspirin, nonsteroidal anti-inflammatory drugs, vitamin E, ginkgo, and other agents that may exacerbate bruising for one week before the procedure.

Multiple approaches exist to counter the anxiety and pain associated with administration of hyaluronic acid fillers. Options include ice, topical anesthesia, field blocks, peripheral nerve blocks, and use of one of the more recently FDA-approved products that intermix anesthesia (lidocaine) into the hyaluronic acid syringe, such as Elevess and Prevelle Silk. Of course, general anesthesia is effective but, unless the patient is requiring general anesthesia for more invasive and coincident procedures, it is the authors' belief that general anesthesia would be excessive. The glabellar area, nasolabial folds, and oral commissures can virtually always be treated using topical anesthetics alone, such as LMX, or combination products, such as topical betacaine, lidocaine, and tetracaine, which can be applied for twenty to thirty minutes before administration to alleviate more sensitive patients and/or treatment areas. However, the clinician should be aware of potential allergic or irritant contact dermatitis stemming from these topical agents. The authors have had success using Pliaglis, a combination topical anesthetic cream of lidocaine and tetracaine, though at the time of this writing it has been discontinued because of its inconsistent viscosity. Particularly painful areas, such as the lips, warrant blocks. Some go so far as to suggest infraorbital and mental nerve blocks with lidocaine to provide sufficient anesthesia for the upper and lower lips, respectively, as well as extended mucosal miniblocks for lateral commissure and surrounding perioral skin.[6] Rarely, some administer oral anxiolytics to relieve the patient of both pretreatment anxiety and concurrent treatment pain. Of note, the application of ice during injections can be very helpful not only in preventing pain but also in minimizing swelling. Easily handled ice applicators can be conveniently produced by freezing small Dixie cups of water overnight. The paper cup may then be peeled away from the ice before use.

Numerous options also exist for the clinician's injection technique. The needle bevel may be directed in any direction, though most prefer to have it up.[2] Studies suggest that the direction does not influence material flow and that instead the hyaluronic acid fillers simply follow the path of least resistance.[2] Appreciation of needle depth is also fundamental to ideal administration, and this often comes with experience. Too deep an insertion into the subcutaneous fat can be recognized since the counter pressure is relatively minimal to that generated by the dermis.[6] On the other hand, too superficial an administration will blanch, dimple, or raise the skin.[6] Typically, the needle is inserted at a thirty- to sixty- degree angle, and the filler contents are injected during withdrawal of the needle. The angle of insertion, however, is highly clinician dependent. The most common injection techniques include linear threading and serial puncture, though fanning and cross-hatching are employed when larger areas, such as the lateral and malar cheek, are being treated.[9] Linear injection involves slow and steady injection while withdrawing the needle along the entire or majority course of treatment area. Serial puncture is similar but instead involves multiple punctures along the line being filled. Fanning also involves injection on retraction, though instead of complete withdrawal of the needle, it is advanced again at a different angle. This can be repeated based on the size of the area being covered. Lastly, cross-hatching involves injections along multiple parallel and perpendicular lines. Whichever technique is employed, it is prudent to reduce and then eliminate product administration as the needle is just leaving the skin to reduce the risk of too superficial placement and consequent nodules. Most experienced injectors feel that they have developed their own particular injection techniques that yield optimal results for their patients.

Many suggest that after injection, the clinician massage the affected area. The intensity and duration of massage, however, are less than that needed for collagen fillers because of hyaluronic acid's greater malleability. Massage is suggested for several reasons. These reasons include the chance to smoothen any uneven product distortions and asymmetries and the chance to modestly rectify any overcorrection. Additionally, an ice pack is typically applied to minimize swelling and to offer mild anesthesia. Lastly, it is good practice to schedule the patient for a follow-up appointment within a few weeks of treatment to fine-tune any incomplete or asymmetric areas as well as to address any patient concerns. Before and after photographs, particularly on the patient's first injection series, are invaluable.

Many other subtleties exist in the application of hyaluronic acid fillers that are beyond the scope of this chapter, including techniques with hyaluronic acids alone and in combination with other filler agents, muscle relaxants, and more. An example of a combination treatment that the authors have used successfully is selective augmentation of the body of the lip with hyaluronic acid filler, subsequently enhanced by collagen injection targeting the vermilion border. Additionally relevant to the practice of hyaluronic acids, though not included in the confines of this chapter, are the array of possibilities with these fillers, including treatment of scars, aging hands, and more.[10]

RISKS ASSOCIATED WITH HYALURONIC ACIDS AND THEIR MANAGEMENT

The use of hyaluronic acids for cosmetic volume enhancement is largely a safe, in-office procedure with high patient satisfaction rates. Adverse reactions generally stem from short-lived hypersensitivity or otherwise local tissue damage inherent to intradermal administration of any product. Another concern, particularly in cases of lip augmentation, includes triggering the recurrence of herpes simplex.[11] For the latter, some clinicians prescribe systemic antivirals when administering hyaluronic acids to patients with a history of recurrent oral herpes labialis. Still, rates of adverse events are very low. In a retrospective study of 262,000 patients treated with Restylane in 2000, 144 patients (0.06 percent) experienced adverse events.[12] Most of these events were short-lived hypersensitivity reactions or injection site inflammation.[12]

Although even rarer, long-term adverse reactions most often involve persistent foreign body–related inflammatory reactions. Since hyaluronic acids are theoretically identical across species and are therefore not antigenic, many propose the foreign body reaction is related to contamination with residual bacterial or animal proteins from the manufacturing process.[11,12] Others suggest that the cross-linkers alone, or the foreign conformations created by cross-linking hyaluronic acids, or their breakdown products are triggering the immunogenic response. Interestingly, recent findings suggest hyaluronic acid may have a direct coregulatory role with activating antigen-presenting cells, T-cells, and macrophages, and this may play a role in these reactions.[11]

Although adverse effects are relatively small in number, many of these effects can be managed by the use of hyaluronidase. Hyaluronidase splits hyaluronic acids at the glucosaminidic bond between C1 of the glucosamine moiety and C4 of glucuronic acid.[13] Although widely used and effective, it remains an off-label use of the product. The enzyme product is derived from mammalian testes, usually ovine or bovine, prompting some clinicians to perform preliminary skin tests.[13] This can be achieved by intradermal injection of small quantities of product with observation for local wheal and flare reaction after five minutes.[13]

Hyaluronidase has proven effective for persistent granulomatous changes described earlier. Other examples of the effectiveness of hyaluronidase for the less common adverse effects are numerous. A recognized adverse effect from hyaluronic acid fillers is a blue–gray discoloration from too superficial injections. This blue appearance is the result of the Tyndall effect. The Tyndall effect stems from wavelengths of light scattering differently based on the substances it encounters and is known among physicists as Rayleigh scattering.[13] Hyaluronidase has proven effective in eliminating the offending hyaluronic acid. It is worth mentioning, however, that an alternative effective treatment for many of these cases includes simple extrusion of the superficial hyaluronic acid through a puncture created by the tip of an eleven-inch blade scalpel or a small needle.[14]

Hyaluronidase has similarly been shown to manage complications in circumstances of excessive product administration and injection necrosis secondary to compression, injury, or vessel obstruction.[13] Therefore, clinicians working with hyaluronic acids would greatly benefit from familiarity with hyaluronidase, and it would be in their best interests to have it readily available.

CONCLUSION

Hyaluronic acid fillers have proven to be a valuable skin augmentation agent. Possessing a favorable safety profile, low allergenicity, and extended longevity, these fillers mitigate degenerative changes by bolstering the underlying connective tissue. Proper technique and appreciation of product differences, however, are fundamental to achieving optimal outcomes. Currently available products are highly effective. Future products hold out the promise of even greater benefits.

REFERENCES

1. Andre P. (2004) Evaluation of the safety of a non-animal stabilized hyaluronic acid (NASHA – Q-Medical, Sweden) in European countries: a retrospective study from 1997 to 2001. *J Eur Acad Dermatol Venereol* **18**, 422–425.

2. Narins RS, et al. (2007) Injectable skin fillers. In: Roenigk RK, et al. (eds.). *Roenigk's Dermatologic Surgery: Current Techniques in Procedural Dermatology.* 3rd ed. (New York, NY: Informa Healthcare) 705.

3. Beddingfield F III, et al. (2008) Fillers in ethnic skin. In: Grimes PE (ed.). *Aesthetics and Cosmetic Surgery for Darker Skin Types.* (Philadelphia, PA: Lippincott, Williams, and Williams) 225.

4. Tezel A, et al. (2008) The science of hyaluronic acid dermal fillers. *J Cosmet Laser Ther* **10**, 35–42.

5. Lupo MP. (2006) Hyaluronic acid fillers in facial rejuvenation. *Semin Cutan Med Surg* **25**, 122–126.

6. Monheit GD, Coleman, KM. (2006) Hyaluronic acid fillers. *Dermatol Ther* **19**, 141–150.

7. Price RD, et al. (2007) Hyaluronic acid: the scientific and clinical evidence. *J Plast Reconstr Aesthet Surg* **60**, 1110–1119.

8. Brandt FS, et al. (2006) Restylane and Perlane. In: Klein AW (ed.). *Tissue Augmentation in Clinical Practice.* (New York, NY: Taylor and Francis) 291.

9. Rohrich RJ, et al. (2007) The role of hyaluronic acid fillers (Restylane) in facial cosmetic surgery: review and technical considerations. *Plast Reconstr Surg* **120**(6S), 41S.

10. Born T. (2006) Hyaluronic acids. *Clin Plast Surg* **33**, 525.

11. Edwards PC, et al. (2007) Review of long-term adverse effects associated with the use of chemically-modified animal and nonanimal source hyaluronic acid dermal fillers. *Clin Interv Aging* **2**, 509.

12. Friedman PM, et al. (2002) Safety data of injectable nonanimal stabilized hyaluronic acid gel for soft tissue augmentation. *Dermatol Surg* **28**, 491.

13. Hirsch RJ, et al. (2007) Hyaluronidase in the office: a necessity for every dermasurgeon that injects hyaluronic acid. *J Cosmet Laser Ther* **9**, 182.

14. Goldman MP, et al. (2006) Soft-tissue augmentation: skin fillers. In: Goldman MP, et al. (eds.). *Advanced Techniques in Dermatologic Surgery.* (New York, NY: Taylor and Francis) 39.

Chapter 5

COLLAGEN PRODUCTS

by

Gary D. Monheit, MD

As collagen has been considered the major building block of dermal structures, it has always been considered an important source for soft tissue injectable implants. Collagen gives support and structural integrity to the skin and associated soft tissue and its loss conversely leads to the thinning and atrophic appearance of both intrinsic and photoaging skin. The triple helical protein structure has a fiber architecture in which intermolecular cross-linking determines the biodurability of collagen in its natural state within the body. The natural balance of collagen degradation and regeneration is upset by UV radiation creating the photodamage that destroys the structure and further leads to dermal loss, facial volume loss, and consequent facial aging[1] (Figure 5.1).

It is no wonder that collagen was early on chosen as a primary substance for all injectable fillers. In the quest for the ideal dermal filler, the following properties were sought:

1. Ease of administration: the product is readily available in a syringe and is easy to inject with good flow characteristics.
2. Physiologic: the product fills the space evenly and is malleable yet remains in place, giving reliable early natural results.
3. No side effects: little or no bruising, edema, inflammation, or other side effects with little chance for prolonged nodules, granulomas, or delayed allergen reactions.
4. Longevity: three months, six months, a year, or permanent have all been named as ideal life spans for filling materials.

Collagen meets many of these criteria, though no material thus far has been found to be perfect.

The science and development of collagen began in 1964 with the identification of its triple helix. In 1968, collagen was first purified, and it was soon discovered by Gross and Kirk that collagen gel could be produced by warming a solution of natural collagen. As collagen subtypes in mammals were identified, it was discovered that autogenic antibodies could be reduced by removing the nonhelical amino acid carboxyl terminal telopeptides[2] (Figure 5.2).

In 1974, the first animal model injections of collagen were given successfully as dermal implants, and in 1978, the first injections of human and bovine collagen were administered into eight patients. These were to correct acne scars, subcutaneous atrophy, and wrinkling. The results demonstrated a 50–80 percent correction of the conditions and were maintained

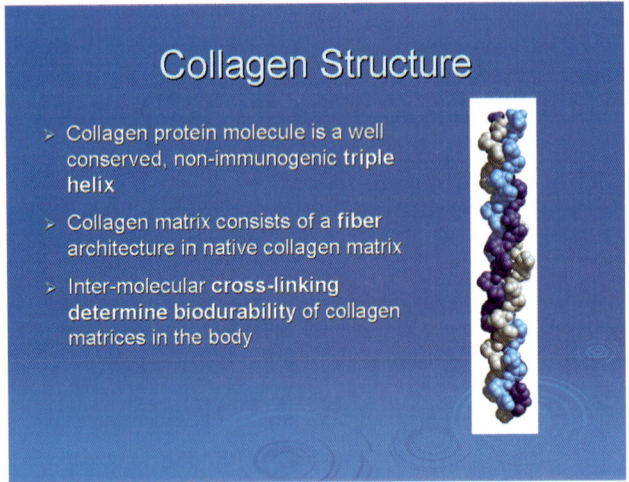

FIG. 5.1. *Collagen structure.*

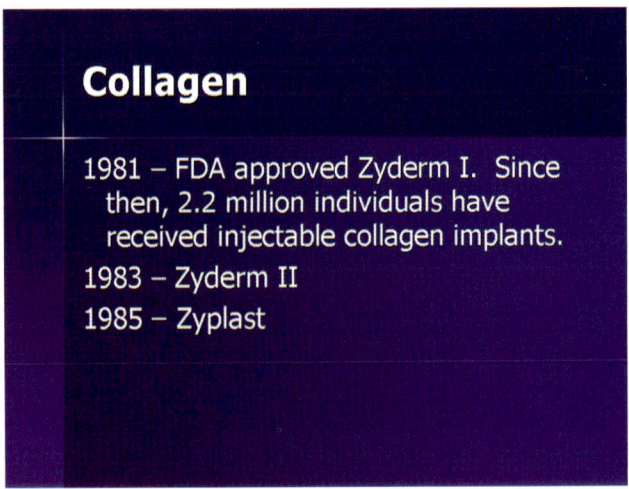

FIG. 5.3. *Collagen.*

up to three months. This was followed by the Tromovitch–Stegman multicenter trial from 1979 to 1980 involving 5,109 subjects using a cross-linked collagen suspension with lidocaine proving both safety and efficacy of the product. In 1981, the FDA approved it for general usage as a dermal filler for the nasolabial fold. Thus, Zyderm I (McGhan Medical, Santa Barbara, CA, later known as Inamed Medical and then Allergan, Irvine, CA) became the first xenogenic agent for soft tissue filling to be followed by two additional formulations of bovine

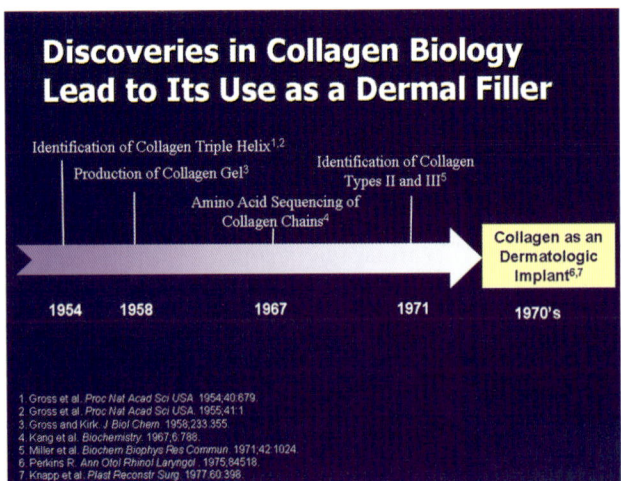

FIG. 5.2. *Discoveries in collagen biology lead to its use as a dermal filler.*

collagen, Zyderm II (1983) and Zyplast (1985).[3] These collagen fillers are xenografts in that they are derived from different animal species (bovine). These products do meet many of the criteria of an ideal soft tissue filling agent as they are ambulatory, reproducible, minimally invasive with little side effects or downtime and predictable efficacy (Figure 5.3).

In the late 1980s, research began on human cadaveric collagens such as Alloderm and Cymetra (Lifecell Corporation, Branchburg, NJ). These are an acellular layer of collagen and elastin derived from cadaveric tissue banks. The products Cymetra and Dermalogen are pulverized and micronized for deep dermal injection to correct depressed acne scars and wrinkles. Because these substances required a large bore needle for injection and created a moderate amount of inflammation, they rapidly lost popularity and presently are not available.

The bovine collagen products rapidly gained popularity, and since then, over 2.5 million individuals have received collagen implants. The products are classified into three types based on viscosity, concentration, and cross-linking (Table 5.1), and all contain lidocaine. All three products may be injected through thirty-gauge needles, though the technique and product placement of each differs.[4]

TABLE 5.1. Collagen Types FDA Approved

Type of Collagen	Concentration of Collagen	Indications	Size of Syringe Available	Placement	Degree of Overcorrection
Zyderm I	35 mg/ml Bovine	Fine lines: perioral, periocular, glabellar	0.5, 1.0, 1.5 cc	Superficial papillary dermis	150–200×
Zyderm II	65 mg/ml Bovine	Mild-moderate rhytids: scars, perioral	0.5, 1.0 cc	Mid-dermis	100–150×
Zyplast	35 mg/ml Cross-linked with glutaraldehyde bovine	Deeper rhytids and folds: nasolabial, vermilion border, marionette lines	1.0, 1.5, 2.0, 2.5 cc	Deep dermis	No overcorrection
Cosmoderm I	35 mg/ml Human derived	Fine lines: perioral, periocular, glabellar	1.0 cc	Superficial papillary dermis	150–200×
Cosmoderm II	65 mg/ml Bovine	Mild-moderate rhytids: Scars, perioral	0.5, 1.0 cc	Mid-dermis	100–150×
Cosmoplast	35 mg/ml Cross-linked with glutaraldehyde, human derived	Deeper rhytids and folds: nasolabial, vermilion border, marionette lines	1.0 cc	Deep dermis	No overcorrection
Evolence	35 mg/ml Cross-linked gel	Deep dermis	0.8 cc	Mid-to-deep dermis	No overcorrection

Skin tests for potential allergic response should be performed before treatment. For the skin test, a 1.0-cc tuberculin syringe with 0.3 ml Zyderm I is used, which screens for all three types. The test should be performed one month before injection, with a second challenge test done two weeks later.[5] A positive test is characterized by swelling, induration, erythema, or pruritus, which can occur in 3 percent of patients indicating a prior bovine collagen allergy. A negative reaction one month after the initial test reduces the risk of hypersensitivity reaction to less than 1 percent.[6]

Because of the need for prior skin testing, a more recent form of human-derived collagen was developed without the need for skin tests and was approved by the FDA in 2003. The three formulations of this human tissue–engineered product are Cosmoderm I, Cosmoderm II, and Cosmoplast corresponding to the bovine products in viscosity but without the need for skin tests[7] (Table 5.1).

Zyderm and Cosmoderm at 35 mg percent can be injected in the superficial dermis or mid-dermis. It is generally used as a superficial filling agent or placed in a layered fashion above the deeper more concentrated products. It requires an overcorrection of up to 150 percent as a significant amount of saline is absorbed. One can appreciate superficial placement by the color blanching of skin or peau d'orange with proper injection (Figure 5.4). Because Zyderm II and Cosmoderm II are 65 mg percent collagen in saline, they do not require overcorrection and are placed in the mid-to-deep dermis. These collagen products will maintain correction for approximately three months after injection. Zyplast and Cosmoplast injectable collagen is different in that the collagen fibers are cross-linked with glutaraldehyde enhancing the product's stability and longevity. It should be injected into the mid-to-deep dermis with no "peau d'orange" and may last longer than the non–cross-linked forms (Figure 5.5).

The collagen implants were the first used to correct skin scars, wrinkles, and folds, and thus, most of our basic injection techniques were developed using these products. Wrinkles and scars amenable for

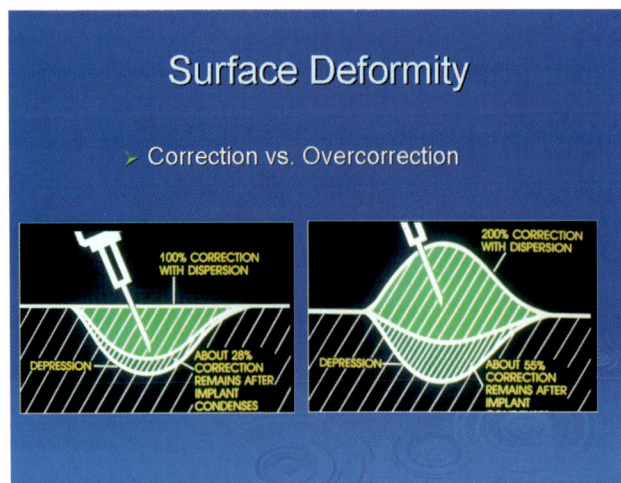

FIG. 5.4. *Surface deformity.*

treatment are distensible, static as opposed to dynamic wrinkles, and not caused by gravitational pull alone. They represent dermal volume depletion, and thus, the lost collagen is most appropriate for replacement. Glabellar lines, forehead wrinkles, and crow's feet have a primary dynamic component that is effectively treated with Botox, but a static component can be treated with the collagens. A primary indication for collagen replacement dermal filling is nasolabial wrinkles and folds, lip wrinkles and lip volume filling, and perioral marionette lines.[7] The success of treatment depends on choosing the appropriate filler for the appropriate patient. To a large

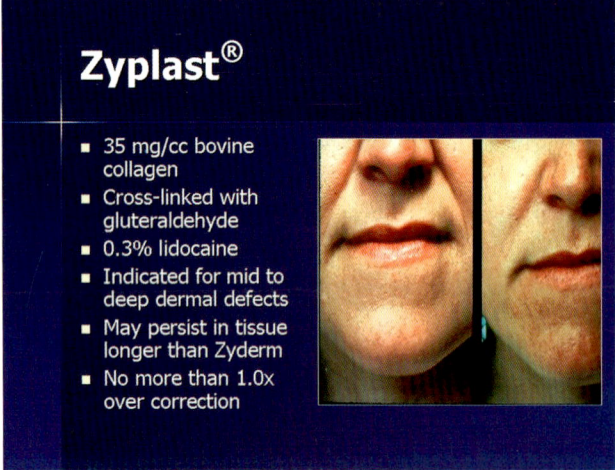

FIG. 5.5. *Zyplast.*

degree, the hyaluronic acid fillers (Restylane, Juvederm) have replaced collagen as volume fillers for lips, deeper folds, and volumizing. The need for collagen still exists for wrinkles and folds and for finer surface lines on the lips and other areas.

Before injections, patients should be taken off blood thinners if possible to minimize bruising and ecchymosis. Bruising is less of a problem using collagen products as opposed to hyaluronic acid fillers that act as anticoagulants. After the skin is thoroughly cleansed and the makeup removed, an alcohol wipe is used to remove residual bacteria. The defect to be corrected such as nasolabial fold is evaluated as to depth and volume of product needed, and the needle is inserted at a forty-five-degree angle, gently releasing the product at the appropriate dermal level for filling. This can be accomplished by serial puncture technique, linear threading, fanning or cross-hatching, or – in the end – a combination of these techniques to create a natural correction. The area is massaged immediately after injection to assure an even distribution of product with no lumpiness, nodules, or beading. Directly after collagen injection, there is very little inflammation, erythema, or induration. In many instances, Zyderm I/Cosmoderm I can be layered over Zyplast/Cosmoplast to give full complete correction. This is especially helpful for lip augmentation, which requires both volume filling with the cross-linked implant and superficial correction of rhagades and the vermilion line that is accomplished with Zyderm I/Cosmoderm I. The results are gratifying for correction of the aging atrophic lip in which collagen will give the filling, support, and superficial correction that is more natural early on than that obtained with hyaluronic acid products.

The goal for correcting an aging atrophic lip is to replace lost volume, further define the vermilion borders, evaluate the oral commissures, and correct vertical rhytids. Volume is usually addressed first by injecting the cross-linked collagen along the vermilion and the "wet–dry" junction of vermilion and mucosa giving both volume filling and elevation. This is best performed via retrograde tunneling or threading technique. The vermilion line is then addressed by injecting laterally within that potential space and "flowing" small amounts of collagen along it maintaining even application and avoiding nodules and overcorrection (Figure 5.6). The obvious "duckbill" or overcorrected upper lip is a deformity and detraction, not a natural correction. The lip should be repeatedly massaged to ensure an even distribution of product with no nodules or beading (Figure 5.7). The oral commissure and marionette line are assessed by pinching the skin together giving an estimation of volume loss and the amount needed to filling the groove and also elevate the depressed commissure. The technique developed for collagen is that which has been maintained for all our fillers involving volume correction of the fold, lower lateral lip, and prejowl crease creating a triangular area of

volume filling, which will act as a wedge to lift the fold and its overhanging prejowl sulcus.

The fold is first filled with Zyplast/Cosmoplast, threading the material to the commissure. A small amount is then injected into the modiolus, which lifts the lateral commissure in a more youthful and

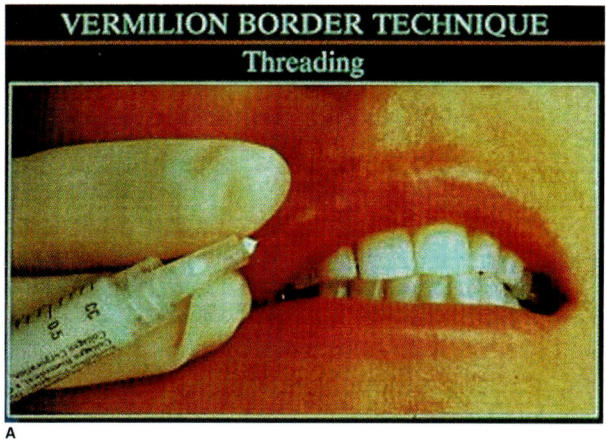

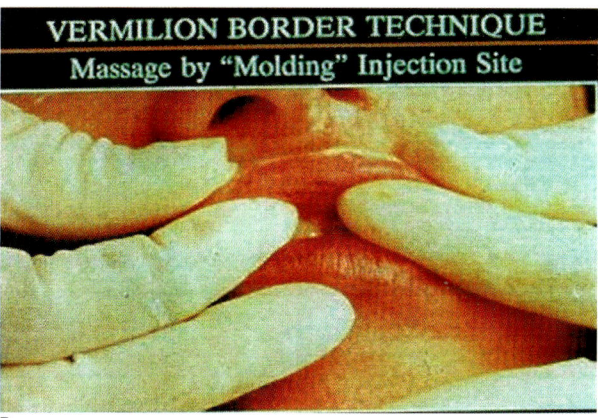

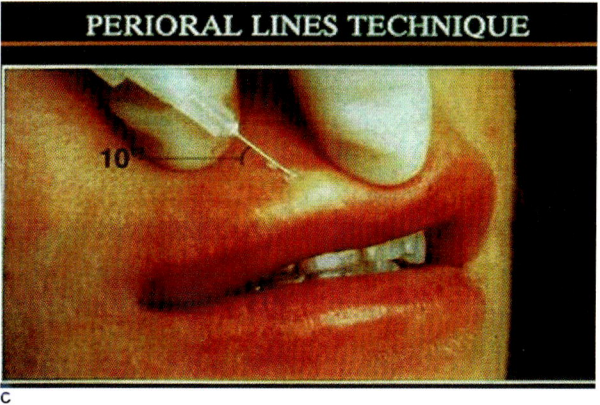

FIG. 5.7. *Lip injection for volume: (A) volume, (B) vermilion shaping, and (C) fine rhytids.*

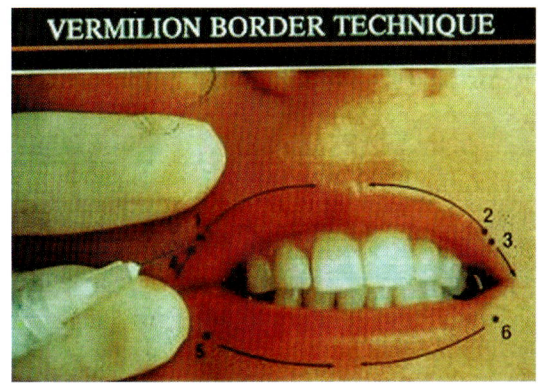

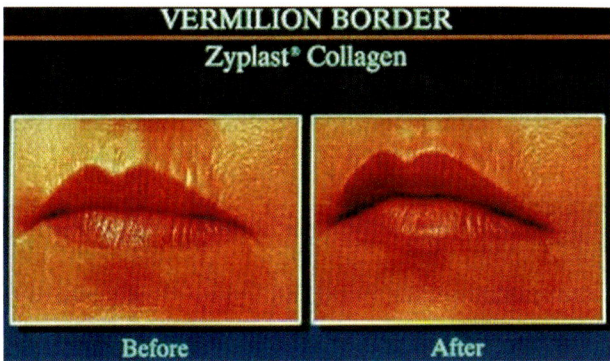

FIG. 5.6. *Threading and serial puncture.*

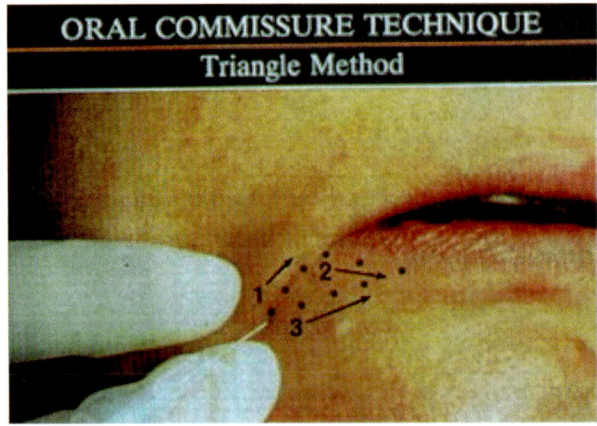

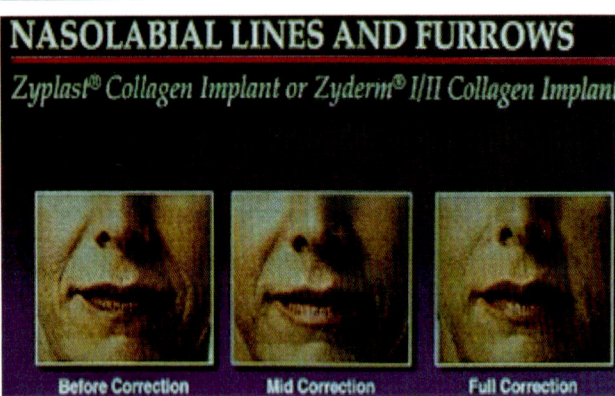

FIG. 5.8.   Oral commissure and marionette lines.

pleasing position. Volume filling of the triangle will add support to lift the overlying lower cheek structure (Figure 5.8).

Finally, the superficial lip components are addressed with the vermilion line, the vertical lines on the upper and lower lip skin, and philtral clefts with the use of Zyderm I or Cosmoderm I layered over the underlying heavier collagen implant. Either threading the lines or serial puncture with immediate massage will give full correction, but care must be taken to use very small volumes in the papillary dermis and it should be massaged immediately.[8]

It is the author's opinion that this combined use of the collagen products determines the most natural lip and perioral correction with least downtime and side effects (Figure 5.9). The disadvantage is longevity as full correction will only last for three to four months. Repeat injection or touch-ups are then needed.

Collagen products can also be used to "top up" dynamic wrinkles already treated with botulinum toxin in which full muscle immobilization is obtained, yet a static wrinkle persists[12] (Figure 5.10). This occurs in the glabellar frown lines, forehead wrinkles, or crow's feet. Zyderm I/Cosmoderm I should only be used for the crow's feet because of the very thin eyelid skin and potential problem of papules or lumpiness. It is also used exclusively for the glabella because of the reported problem or vascular infarction with the cross-linked products. This occurs with the heavier products injected deeply in this area where larger vessels can be injected causing

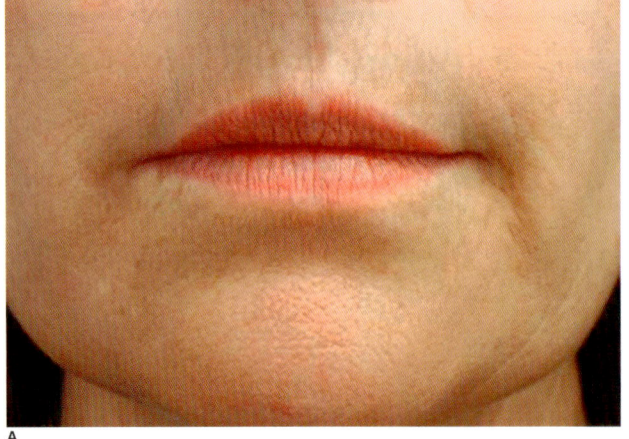

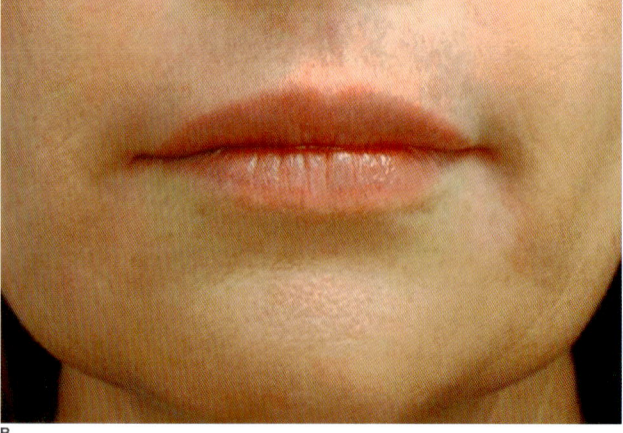

FIG. 5.9.   Zyplast with Zyderm layered above: (A) before and (B) after.

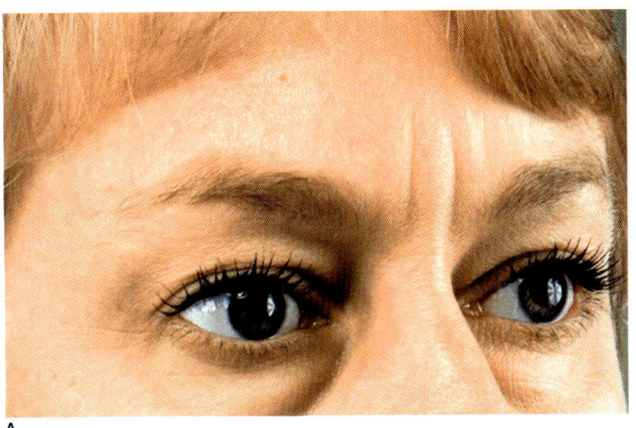
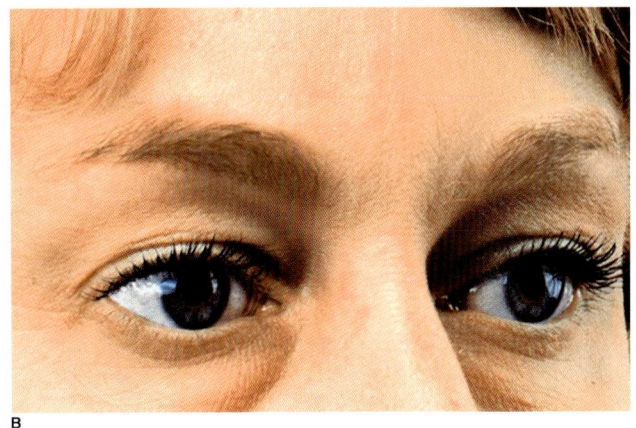

A | B

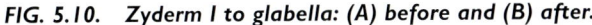

FIG. 5.10. *Zyderm I to glabella: (A) before and (B) after.*

infarction and thus skin sloughing. This can also occur at the superior triangle of the nasolabial fold where the angular artery can be injected. The first sign of infarction is a surrounding blanching of skin. At that point, the injection should be stopped and the area massaged vigorously. If the blanching persists, the area can be treated with nitroglycerine paste and Acetyl-Salicylic Acid (ASA) Grade V given orally as an anticoagulant. Most cases resolve promptly with treatment before the development of skin necrosis, sloughing, and finally scar formation.[9]

It has been twenty-five years since the first collagen fillers were released, and they still are used effectively. Their popularity though has been greatly diminished by the release of the more versatile and longer lasting hyaluronic acid fillers. It is the author's opinion, though there is still a place for collagen injectable filling material and hope our only supplier will continue to keep the products in the commercial market (Figure 5.11).

The need for a longer lasting, less immunogenic yet robust dermal filler has led to the development of a new porcine-based dermal filler, Evolence. This was developed in Haifa, Israel, by Colbar Corporation, now a division of Johnson and Johnson. Rather than using mixed dermal collagen (types I, II, and III), this product uses only type I collagen harvested from porcine Achilles tendon. Type I collagen forms the largest and strongest of fibers making it ideal for implants and other medical devices including heart valve replacements, corneal shields, wound dressings, and surgical meshes for tissue repair. The fibers are digested with pepsin for separation to monomeric collagen fibers, and the immunogenic telopeptides are removed eliminating the risk of xenogenic allergy. The fillers are then polymerized as reconstituted polymeric collagen. The polymeric collagen is then cross-linked with ribose producing Evolence collagen. This "glymatrix" process of cross-linking is unique to fillers in that the sugar has no toxicity, and thus, larger amounts are used than found with glutaraldehyde, BDDE, or other cross-linkers that are potentially toxic and used sparingly by FDA safety parameters. The glymatrix technology creates a longer lasting, more robust product that can provide correction for up to one year (Table 5.2). Evolence has been used in Europe for over five years with success as a facial wrinkle and groove filler with little reported side effects or complications.[10] Evolence is used for moderate-to-deep wrinkles and injected in the deep dermis with a twenty-seven-gauge needle. It is effective for correction of nasolabial folds and marionette lines. Evolence does have a thinner, more refined companion product – Evolence Breeze – which is intended for more superficial placement and lip

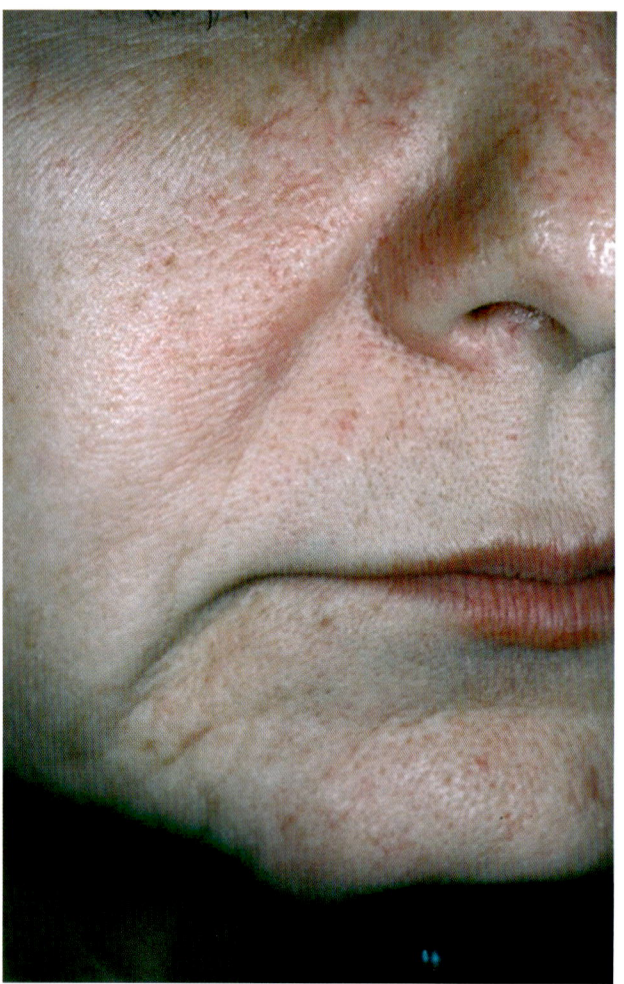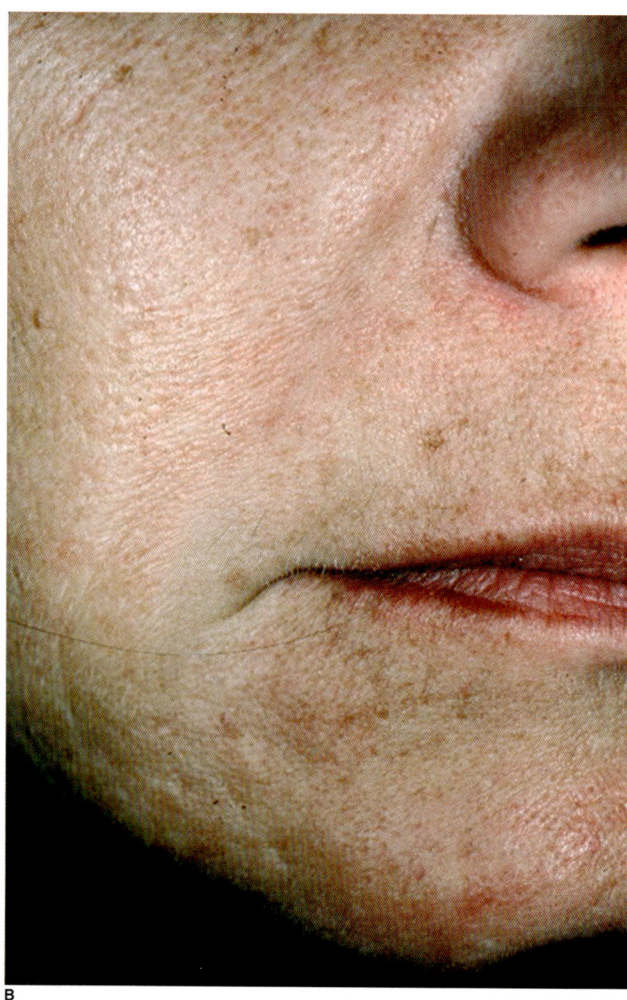

FIG. 5.11.   Cosmoplast to nasolabial fold: (A) before and (B) after.

filling. Evolence Breeze is injected through a thirty-gauge needle in the mid-dermis. Both products are different from their bovine collagen predecessors, and the technique of injection is thus different (Figure 5.12). Evolence should be injected with a linear threading technique with a slow, steady injection and

no overcorrection. It was FDA approved in June 2008 and released in the open market in September 2008. Evolence Breeze is not FDA approved but is available in Europe and in Canada.

Evolence has been thoroughly studied for hypersensitivity with skin test and antibody studies that

TABLE 5.2. Glymatrix Technology

	Glymatrix™	Other
Biomaterial	Collagen	Vary (e.g., collagen, hyaluronic acid)
Cross-linking material	Natural sugar	Chemicals: fixatives (formalin, glutaraldehyde, etc.)
Cross-linking degree	Controlled – producing programmed biomaterials	Limited – either due to toxicity or adverse reaction
Durability	Enhanced at least 12 months	Limited 3–9 months
Matrix properties	Mimics skin's three-dimensional matrix, both structurally and functionally	Altered biologic properties

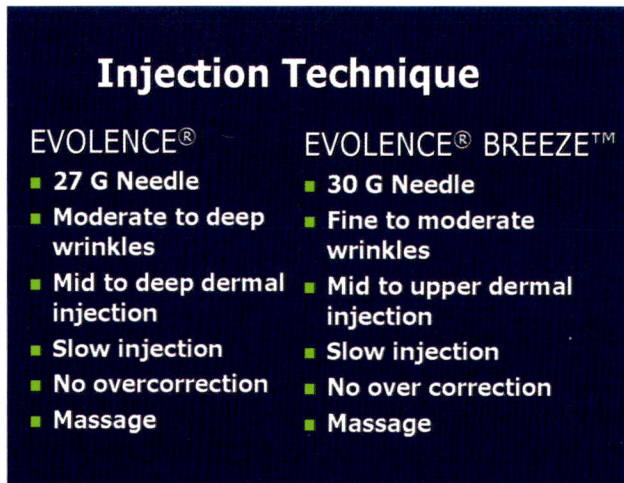

FIG. 5.12. *Injection technique.*

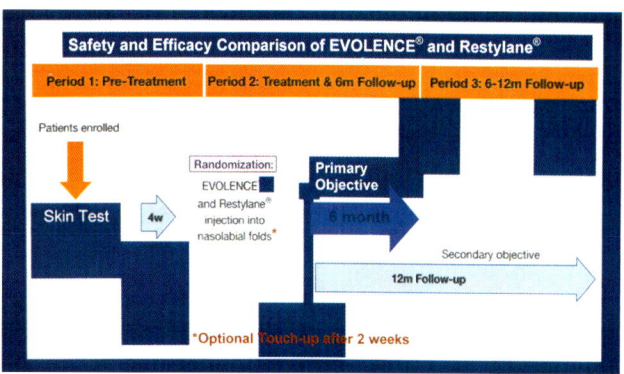

FIG. 5.13. *Pivotal study (DP101 US-01): study design.*

confirmed its safety so that no skin test is required.[11] Multiple biopsy studies in animal models and humans confirm the good tissue integration and host response with demonstrable evidence of fibroblastic activity and neocollagenesis. Evolence has further benefits in that it is nonhydrophilic, which minimizes swelling, and also is hemostatic minimizing bruising and bleeding. It thus offers predictable correction with little downtime.[12]

Contraindications and precautions include hypersensitivity reactions to collagen, patients with bleeding disorders, or those with compromised immune function. The product is tested and indicated for injection into the dermis of the face, and care should be taken to avoid blood vessels because of vascular occlusion and subsequent necrosis, especially in the glabella.

The pivotal FDA study for Evolence was a double-blind, within-subject bilateral facial comparison of Evolence versus Restylane for the correction of nasolabial folds. Its evaluation was for efficacy, safety, and longevity. Testing was conducted at six investigator sites with principal investigators: Rhoda Narins, MD, and Gary Monheit, MD[13] (Figure 5.13).

Subjects were selected with moderate-to-deep nasolabial folds on the modified Fitzpatrick wrinkle scale (2 or greater) and up to two injections were used to correct both folds: One with Evolence and the other with Restylane. The subjects were followed for six months initially and then for a year for efficacy and safety. Although the product has been used with no clinical allergic reactions, skin tests as well as sequential antibody levels were performed and followed throughout the study. The results from immunoglobulin titers and skin tests indicated no potential for allergic reactions and the FDA did in fact release the product without the need for prior skin testing.

The data from the initial six months of the study indicated no meaningful difference between the Evolence treatment sides and the Restylane-treated nasolabial folds at any point (Figure 5.14). Patient evaluation also indicated a 90 percent improvement over baseline at six months on both sides. In addition, the safety profiles were similar for both with no significant reaction. The reaction of induration, swelling, bruising, and pain was higher on the NASHA treatment side (Figure 5.15).

The study thus demonstrated noninferiority to HA in the correction of nasolabial folds at six months with a 90 percent report of patient satisfaction as compared to baseline.

Of the 148 subjects followed for six months, 145 patients were followed for efficacy and safety for an additional twelve months. Filler persistence or a wrinkle severity score of 1 over baseline was maintained at

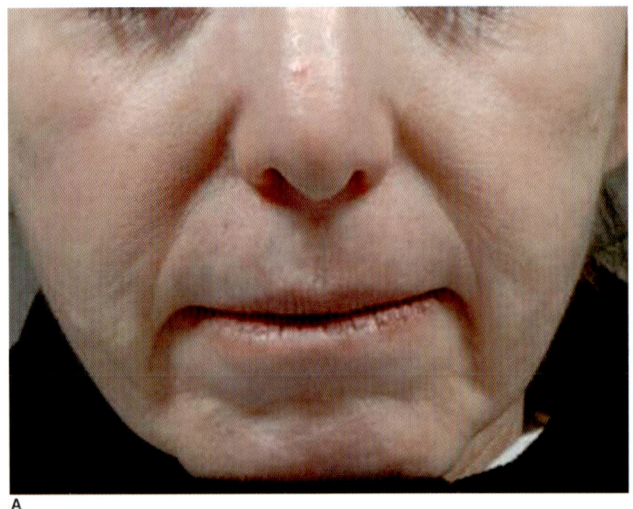
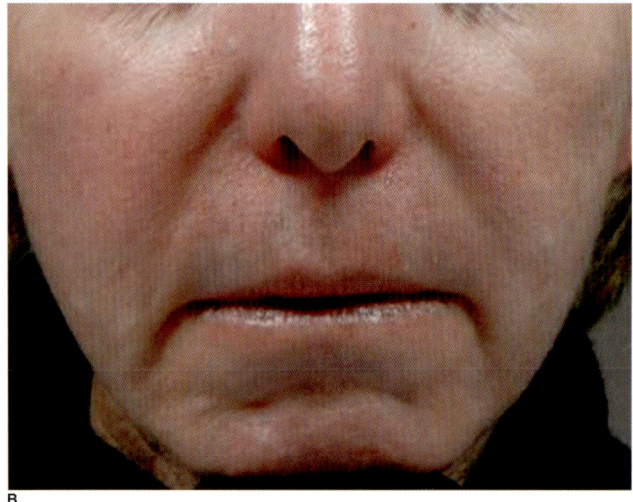

FIG. 5.14.   (A) Before treatment and (B) after treatment (see Figure 5.12).

twelve months in 75 percent of the subjects. In addition, long-term safety was good with no delayed granulomas or infections.[14,15]

USE

Evolence is supplied in a 1-ml syringe with a twenty-seven-gauge needle. The recommended treatment protocol is a mid-to-deep dermal injection using antero- or retrograde tunneling technique. The slow continuous flow of the product during injection will give an even distribution of the implant through the area to be corrected. After and during injection, the implant should be massaged to ensure even correction to prevent the formation of papules or nodules. This collagen "sets up" quickly, and if the product is injected too quickly or with stops and starts, it will be lumpy and will produce nodules. Overcorrection in any area is not recommended as it will remain if not vigorously massaged early on (Figure 5.16).

As one evaluates a patient for injection, volume for correction should be estimated, which will relate to the number of syringes needed. There is no lidocaine in the product so that adequate local or topical anesthesia is needed. Some of the topical "caine" mixtures may suffice for nasolabial fold injections or patients can have an infraorbital and/or mental

nerve block for full local anesthesia. Makeup should be removed, and the area should be cleaned thoroughly with alcohol wipes. The product is stored at room temperature and in fact should be warmed between hands before injection. A cold product may clog the needle or clump up within the skin. This is further reason to abstain from the use of ice with Evolence for pre- or postinjection. The needle is tightly affixed to the luer lock and the product should be used immediately after assembling and priming the syringe and needle. One should inject at a slow and steady pace without interruption. This product flows more easily and smoothly than many HAs, so less pressure should be used on the plunger to give that slow even flow.

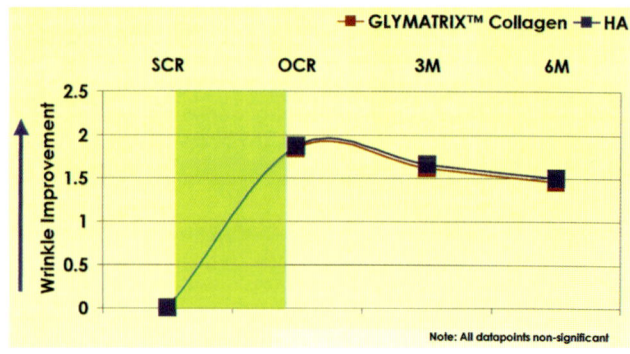

FIG. 5.15.   Improvement in wrinkle.

FIG. 5.16. *Evolence to nasolabial fold: (A) preinjection, (B) thirty to sixty minutes, and (C) twelve to sixteen hours postinjection.*

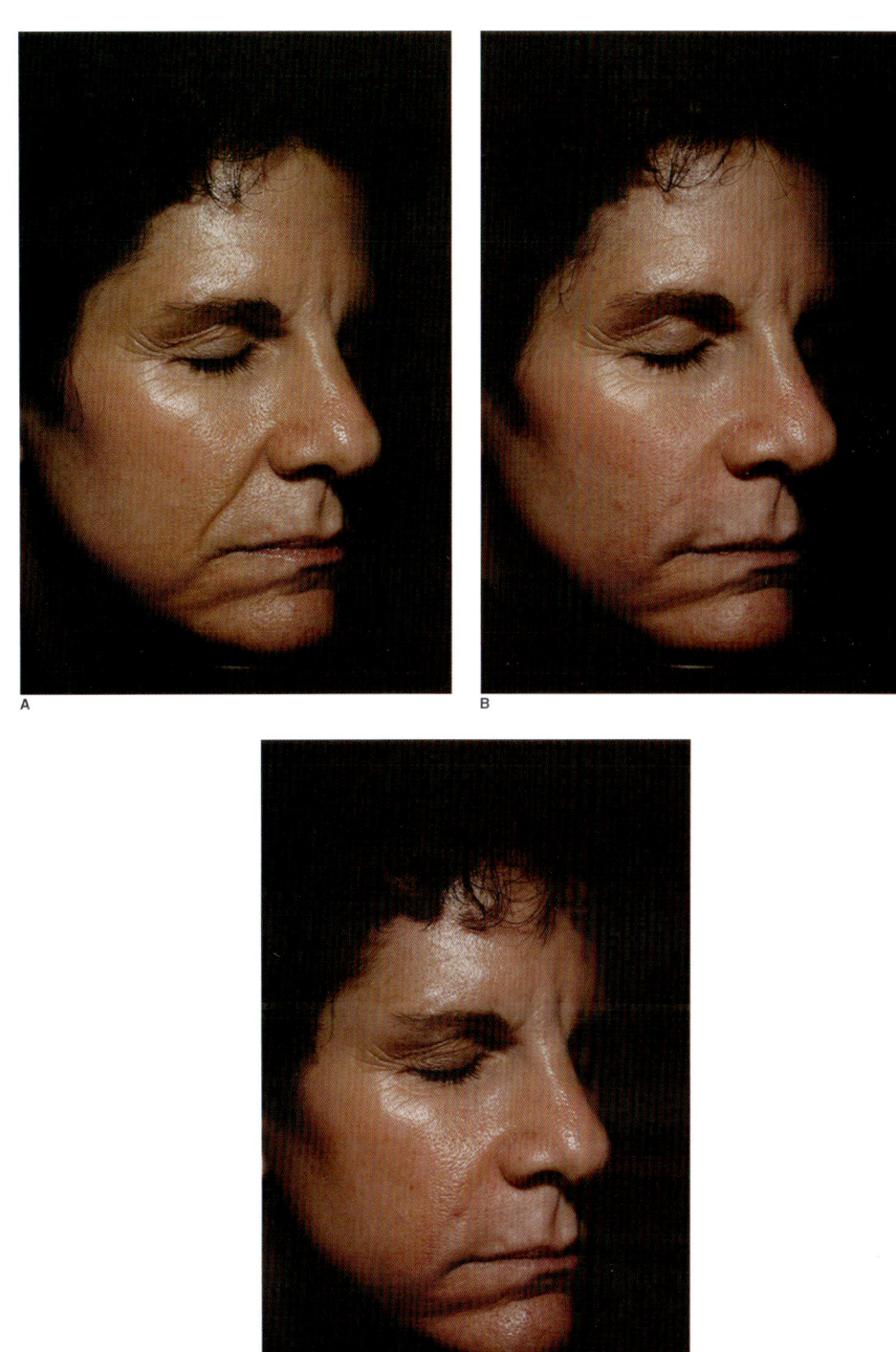

Immediately after injection, gentle massage is needed to remodel and sculpt the injected area and also to palpate for any papules or bumps. This should be done immediately as the product will set up quickly. Once done, the product will not migrate.

Undesired problems that can occur are generally those that appear with most fillers. These include pain

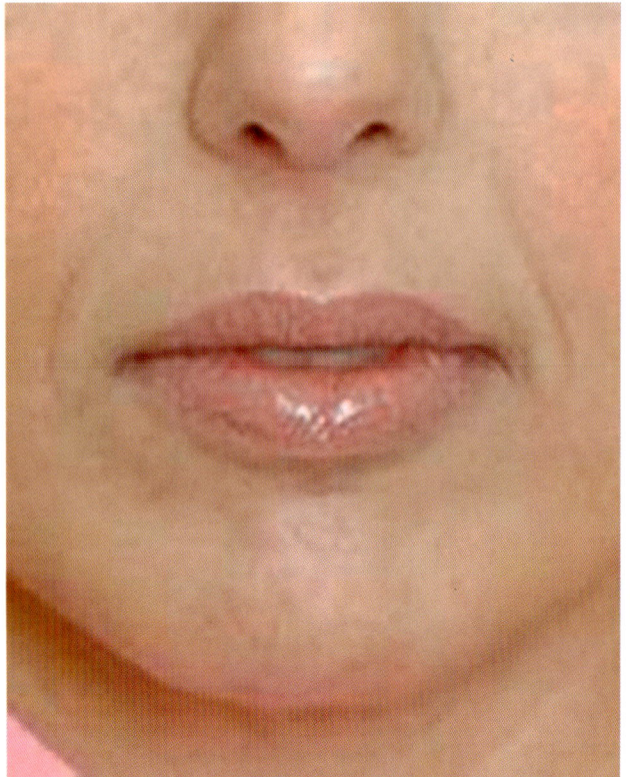
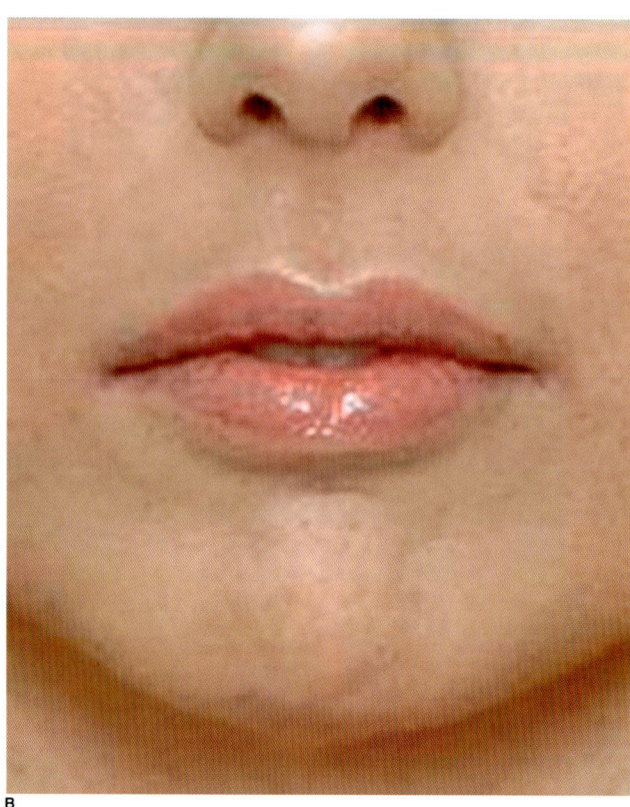

A   **B**

FIG. 5.17.   Nasolabial lines treated with Evolence – 30 (A) before and (B) after.

on injection, erythema, edema, ecchymosis, and urticaria. Of especial concern are the embolism, ulceration, and necrosis that can occur with injection in an artery. It is thus not indicated in the glabellar region as other cross-linked collagen fillers have been restricted. Nodularity and postinjection bumps are an unwanted problem and have been seen with Evolence injected into the lips. The product thus should not be used as a lip filler. Evolence Breeze, which is not yet available in the United States, will be the collagen product for lip use. Nodules and papules can be avoided with good injection technique and appropriate placement of the product in the mid-to-deep dermis.

If a nodule is present after twenty-four hours, it may be difficult to eradicate. One can try saline injection to break up the collagen fibers or conservative use of diluted triamcinolone acetamide (2.5 mg percent in saline). Overuse of steroid injection will produce atrophy in surrounding skin making the situation worse.

Evolence thus has a real value in our armamentarium of dermal fillers as a longer lasting collagen delivering good correction with immediate results and minimal downtime (Figure 5.17). The further Evolence Breeze product will be an addition for use in lips and more superficial filling.

Collagen products were the first injectable implant for use in the United States and today remain the mainstay for dermal filling. It replaces aging and atrophic collagen in photoaging skin and gives a very natural, predictable correction. Whether bovine, synthetically human based, or porcine, the collagen family will remain an important tool for treatment of the aging face.

REFERENCES

1. Hanke CW, Coleman WP. Collagen filler substances. In Coleman WP, Hanke CW, Alt TH, Askin S (eds.).

Cosmetic Surgery of the Skin: Principles and Techniques. Philadelphia; BC Decker 1991:89–102.

2. McPherson JM, et al. The preparation and physio-chemical characterization of an injectable form of reconstituted, glutaraldehyde cross-linked, bovine corium collagen. *J Biomed Meter Res* 1986; **20**:79–92.

3. Castrow FF II, Krull EA. Injectable collagen implant-update. *J Am Acad Dermatol* 1983; **9**:889–893.

4. Matarasso SL. The use of injectable collagen for aesthetic rejuvenation. *Semin Cutan Med Surg* 2006; **25**:151–157.

5. Elson ML. The role of skin testing in the use of collagen injectable materials. *J Dermatol Surg Oncol* 1989; **15**:301–303.

6. Klein AW. In favor of double testing. *J Dermatol Surg Oncol* 1989; **15**:263.

7. Matarasso SL, Sadick NS. Soft tissue augmentation. In Bolognia J, Jorizzo JL, Rapini RV, Horn T (eds.). *Dermatology*. London; Mosby, Harcourt Health Sciences; 2439–2449.

8. Kaminer MS, Kraus MC. Filler substance in the treatment of facial aging. *Med Surg Dermatol* 1998; **15**: 215–222.

9. DeBoule K. Management of complications after implantation of fillers. *J Cosmet Dermatol* 2004; **3**(1): 2–15.

10. Monstrey SJ, Pitrau S, Hamdi M, et al. A two stage phase I trial of Evolence collagen for soft tissue contour correction. *Plast Reconstr Surg* 2007; **120**:303–311.

11. Shoshani D, Markovitz E, Cohen Y, et al. A skin test hypersensitivity study of a cross-linked porcine collagen implant for aesthetic surgery. *Dermatol Surg* 2007; **33**:S152–S158.

12. Pitrau S, Noff M, Blok L, et al. Long term efficacy of a novel ribose-cross-linked collagen dermal filler: a histo-logic and histomorphometric study in an animal model. *Dermatol Surg* 2007; **53**:1–10.

13. Narins R, et al. A randomized multicenter study of the safety and efficacy of dermicil-P35 and non-animal stabilized hyaluronic acid gel for the correction of nasolabial folds. *Dermatol Surg* 2007; **33**:S213–S221.

14. Narins R, Monheit G, et al. One year follow up study of Evolence for the correction of nasolabial folds. Presentation at the World Congress of Dermatology, Buenos Aires, September 24, 2007.

15. Narins RS, Brandt FS, Lorenc ZP, Maas CS, Monheit GD, Smith SR. Twelve month persistency of a novel ribbons-cross-linked collagen dermal filler. *Dermatol Surg* 2008; **34**(supp 1):S31–S39.

Chapter 6

RADIESSE

by

Neil S. Sadick, MD

INTRODUCTION

Synthetic particulate-based materials are notable for their ability to provide a robust and durable implant and have long been used as bulking agents in a variety of surgical and nonsurgical settings. Radiesse® (BioForm Medical, Inc., San Mateo, CA) is an injectable filler material composed of synthetic calcium hydroxylapatite (CaHA) microspheres suspended in an aqueous carrier gel. Seventy percent of the composition of Radiesse is sodium carboxymethylcellulose carrier gel; the remaining 30 percent of the composition is CaHA microspheres. These uniform microspheres (25–45 microns) are identical in composition to the mineral portion of human bone and teeth.[1–3]

CaHA has been used for over twenty years in various forms in plastic and reconstructive surgery, otology, otolaryngology, neurosurgery, orthopedic surgery, maxillofacial surgery, and dentistry.[4] The excipients that comprise the aqueous gel carrier (i.e., cellulose, glycerin, and sterile water) are classified as "Generally Recognized as Safe" (21 CFR 182) by the Food and Drug Administration and have an extensive record of use in intramuscular injectable products such as Cortone®, Decadron®, and Dalalone®.[2]

The components of CaHA occur naturally in the body and therefore are inherently biocompatible. Results from extensive in vitro and in vivo safety studies, including toxicology assessments, standardized biocompatibility testing, and a three-year animal study, demonstrate that injectable CaHA is biocompatible, nontoxic, nonirritating, and nonantigenic.[2] Because CaHA contains no animal or human tissue derivatives, patient sensitivity testing is not required before use.[2]

In the United States, injectable CaHA has been used for several years for correction of oral/maxillofacial defects, vocal fold augmentation, and as a radiographic tissue marker. A formulation with larger CaHA microspheres, Coaptite®, is approved as a bulking agent in treatment of stress urinary incontinence.[5,6]

In 2006, Radiesse received FDA approval for correction of facial fat loss (lipoatrophy) in patients with human immunodeficiency virus (HIV), based on results of an eighteen-month open-label trial.[7] It is also approved for correction of moderate-to-deep lines and folds, such as nasolabial folds (NLFs), based on results of a comparative pivotal trial.[8] In this trial, 117 patients received injections of CaHA in one NLF and human collagen (Cosmoplast®, Allergan) in the other. At six months, significantly more patients who received CaHA (82 percent) showed improvement compared to control (27 percent) ($P < 0.001$).[8] Its use in a variety of off-label aesthetic applications has also been reported in the literature. Lower face uses include correction of moderate-to-deep creases, such as the oral commissure, marionette lines, mental crease, lateral chin, and prejowl sulcus. Midface uses include volume augmentation in the malar, submalar, and infraorbital regions and nose.[3,9–16]

MECHANISM OF ACTION

After injection, the carrier gel is gradually absorbed, and the CaHA particles remain. A local fibroblastic response at the site results in collagen matrix encapsulation of the CaHA particles, similar to a grapevine growing through a garden trellis (Figure 6.1). The result is a highly biocompatible long-lasting implant with similar characteristics to adjacent tissue. Thus, when CaHA is implanted in soft tissue, new soft tissue develops.[17] No calcification or osteogenesis has been reported in the extensive literature describing the use of CaHA in a variety of soft tissue applications.[1,18,19]

A study of dermal tissue biopsies after injection of Radiesse, light microscopy, and electron microscopy at one month postinjection revealed the presence of CaHA microspheres, with minimal or no inflammatory response or fibrosis.[17] Histologic analysis at

six months postinjection showed tight aggregates of CaHA microspheres with extracellular matrix replacement of gel. Electron microscopy studies demonstrated an increase in histiocytes and associated fibroblasts, which appear to anchor down the microspheres and encourage new collagen formation.[17] The persistence of microspheres and new tissue formation observed was accompanied by evidence of clinical improvement at six months. From a safety perspective, it is important to note that there was no evidence of granuloma formation, ossification, or foreign body reactions at one or six months (Figure 6.2).[17]

Durability

Over time, the CaHA particles are metabolized and removed through normal homeostatic pathways. In one long-term animal study, CaHA particles remained intact at the site of injection throughout the entire three-year study period.[20] Studies in humans have not shown three-year durability but have shown results that extended past the twelve-month

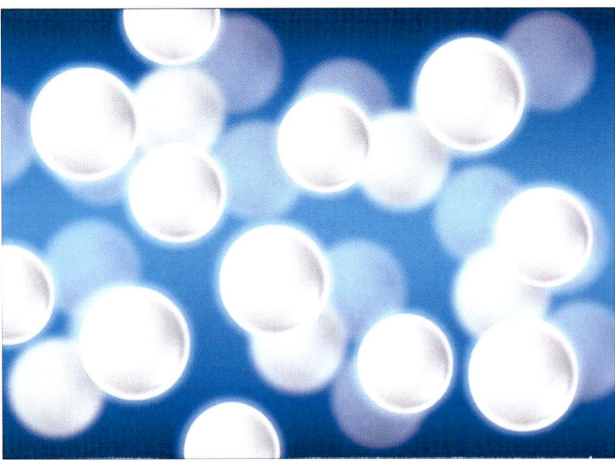

FIG. 6.1. *CaHA microspheres, 25–45 micron diameter. (Illustration courtesy of BioForm Medical, Inc.)*

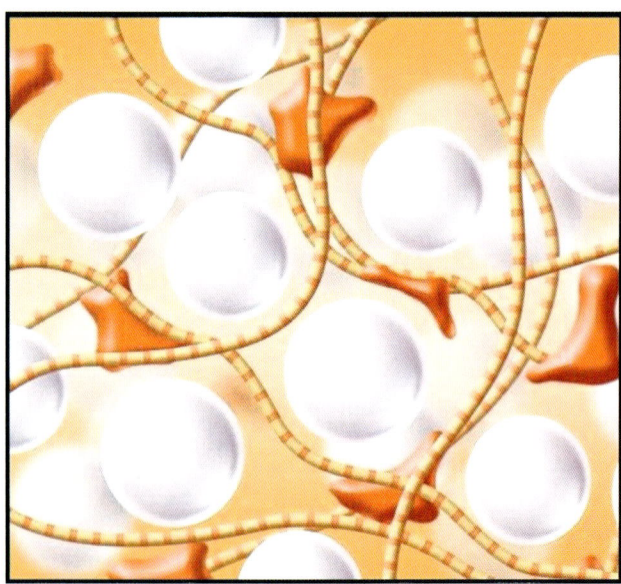

FIG. 6.2. *CaHA in soft tissue, with collagen infiltration. (Illustration courtesy of BioForm Medical, Inc.)*

mark. In vivo, the durability of CaHA can be expected to vary depending on such factors as injection technique, site of material placement, and patient age and metabolism. The longevity of aesthetic correction in the face has been reported to range from ten to fourteen months with an average correction of one year.[9,16] Other sources report longevity of correction of twelve to eighteen months.[1,3,18,21]

AESTHETIC APPLICATIONS

Treatment sites amenable to CaHA injection include the NLFs, marionette lines (melolabial folds), perioral lines, prejowl sulcus, zygoma and malar eminence, tear trough depressions, nose, and acne scars (Figure 6.3).

THE PROCEDURE

Equipment and Patient Preparation

The patient should first be counseled about what to expect in terms of any discomfort that may occur during or after injection, possible side effects, the results that he or she can expect, and the likely durability of correction. Informed consent should be obtained. It is strongly recommended that pretreatment and posttreatment photographs be taken; comparing pretreatment and posttreatment photographs may help patients more objectively evaluate their results.

Before beginning the procedure, the injection site should be identified with a washable marker. For best results, the patient should be seated upright to account for the effects of gravity. Pretreatment photographs should be taken after the marking. The equipment tray should be set up so that the injecting clinician has both equipment and soft tissue filler easily at hand.

Radiesse requires no special handling or storage considerations. It may be stored at room temperature for up to two years. Radiesse syringes are intended

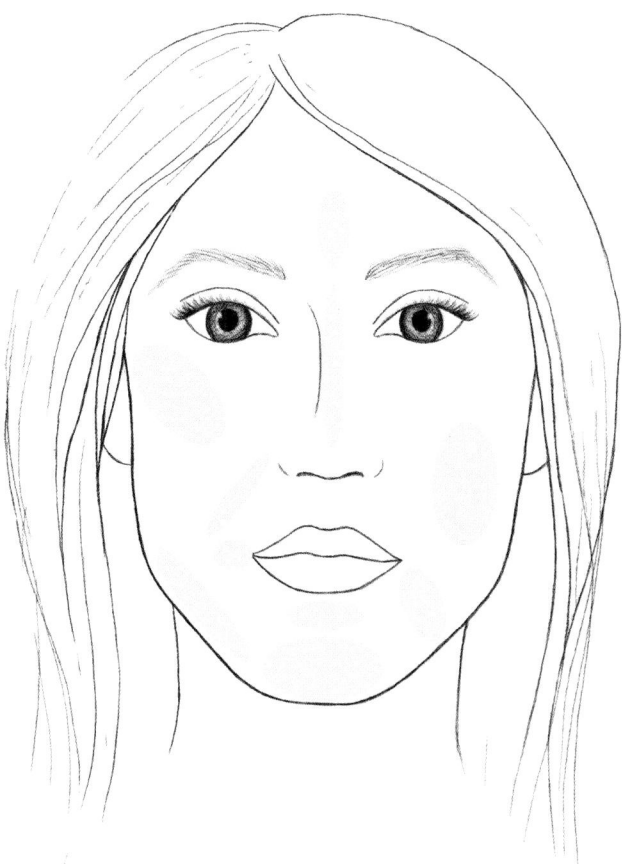

FIG. 6.3. *Areas of treatment with Radiesse. (Illustration courtesy of BioForm Medical, Inc.)*

to be single use only; all unused material should be discarded.

Technique and Aesthetic Considerations

CaHA provides immediate and long-lasting cosmetic correction. The material is versatile in that it may be used to correct soft tissue deficiencies as well as enhance areas of skeletal resorption as occurs with age (e.g., malar and infraorbital areas). The correction is approximately 1:1 and is apparent immediately upon injection. Overcorrection is not necessary, nor is there a need to build correction over multiple sessions. Some clinicians feel that performing a refinement of areas augmented at two to three months postinjection extends the duration of correction; others do not routinely administer these additional injections, preferring instead to generate full correction on the initial visit.

CaHA is typically injected using a twenty-seven-gauge ½- or 1¼-inch needle. It should be injected in a retrograde fashion using a linear, threading, fanning, and/or cross-hatching technique, depending on the area being treated.

Injection volumes vary with the treatment site. Generally, a lesser volume of CaHA is required to provide the same degree of correction as hyaluronic acid and collagen. This observation is confirmed by data from two studies of Radiesse in the NLFs: In these studies, a single syringe of Radiesse was shown to provide better correction than a syringe of Cosmoplast, Restylane, Perlane, or Juvederm.[8,22,23]

Depth of injection for Radiesse is dependent on the area being augmented and the desired effect. In areas where line filling is desired, such as in the NLFs or marionette lines, Radiesse is placed in the deep dermis to subdermal plane. In contrast, where restoring volume is desired, such as the midface, Radiesse is best placed in the subcutaneous space to provide for a filling and lifting over a larger surface area.

Nasolabial Folds

Radiesse is our preferred filler for this area because it can be injected deep at the level of the subdermal plane and because it provides relative durability despite the dynamic motion of this area.

Prior to injection, local anesthesia may be administered using Xylocaine (1 percent) or lidocaine (1 percent) with 1:100,000 epinephrine. To reduce tissue edema and ecchymosis, ice packs may be applied before and after injections.

In treating the NLFs, a fine linear threading technique should be used to deposit the filler in strands of approximately 0.05 mL per pass into the subdermal plane medial to the skin fold and at the depth of the skin crease, bringing the deficiency to full correction. No overcorrection is required (Figure 6.4).

The injection area should be gently molded by the physician and shaped for smoothness immediately after injection using a bidigital technique, followed by application of an ice pack to aid in reducing edema and ecchymosis. Patients should be observed for any adverse reactions and counseled about the need to contact their physician post-treatment, should a severe adverse reaction occur (Figure 6.5A,B).

Marionette Lines

Marionette lines are more resistant to correction with any filler and may prove more difficult to correct completely, presumably due to the dynamic motion of this area. After local injection of lidocaine, Radiesse may be injected subdermally to create a foundation of material, following by linear passes and cross-hatching within the deep dermis to layer additional material (Figures 6.6 and 6.7A,B).[1]

Care should be taken to remain conservative in the volumes placed in this area as overzealous

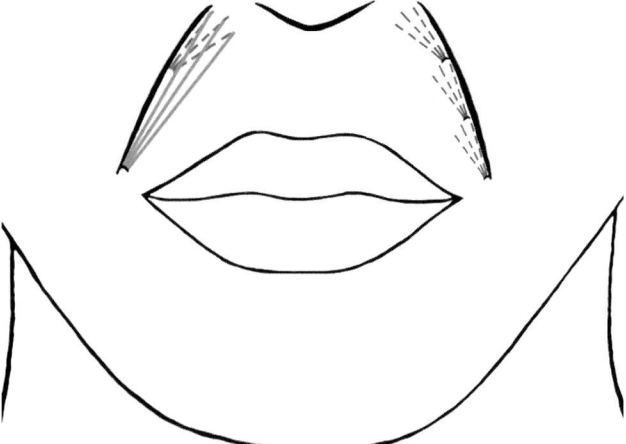

FIG. 6.4. *Linear and fanning techniques in the area of the NLFs. (Illustration courtesy of BioForm Medical, Inc.)*

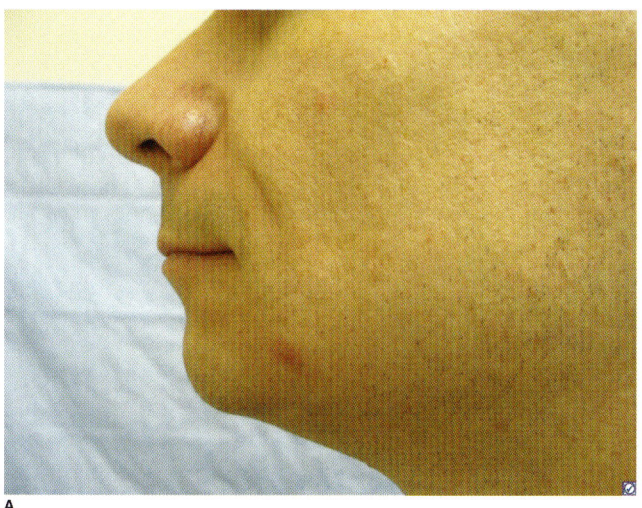
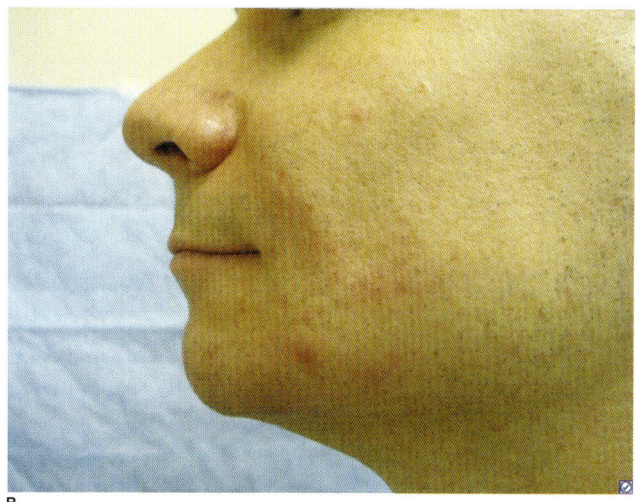

A

B

FIG. 6.5. *(A) Patient before injection into the NLFs. (B) Patient immediately after injection into the NLFs.*

placement of material may lead to accumulation on the mucosal surface of the oral cavity.

Malar Augmentation

In addition to filling creases and other defects, Radiesse may be used for volume augmentation in areas such as the cheeks. Cheek augmentation is increasing in popularity as an application for fillers because of its rejuvenating effect on the face as a whole. Radiesse is often chosen for malar enhance-

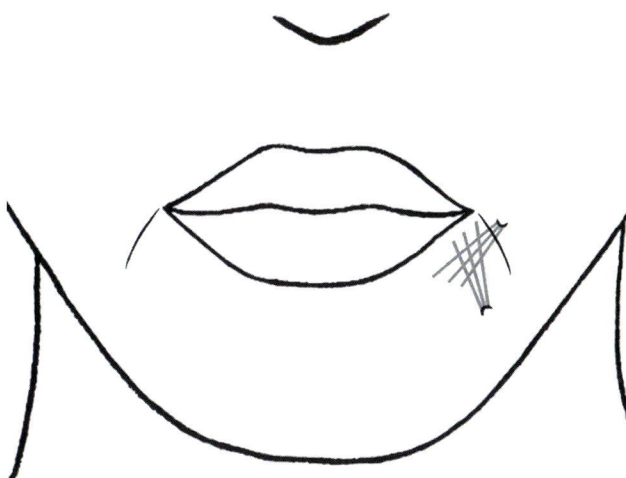

FIG. 6.6. *Threading and cross-hatching in the area of the marionette lines. (Illustration courtesy of BioForm Medical, Inc.)*

ment because of its durability, its volumizing property, and its structural integrity.

When treating multiple areas, malar/submalar augmentation should be performed first because augmentation often affects other areas of the face. In particular, augmentation of the malar and midface areas may lessen the volume of material required for NLF correction by taking up excess skin and lifting the midface region as a whole.

To enhance patient comfort during malar injection, administration of an infraorbital nerve block is recommended. This can be accomplished using only a relatively small amount of anesthetic, 0.2–0.3 mL per side, followed by massage. A local anesthetic should be applied directly into the tissue along the lateral aspect of the zygoma to ensure patient comfort throughout the facial contouring procedure.

Our preferred technique for malar augmentation is to use insertion points at the NLF and zygoma and then proceed upward with injection into the submalar soft tissue, layering three-dimensional, multiple linear threads in a fanning motion across the malar eminence. Cross-hatching of material in multiple planes and depths provides for optimal structural support. The threading pattern into the malar area roughly approximates the shape of an inverted right triangle

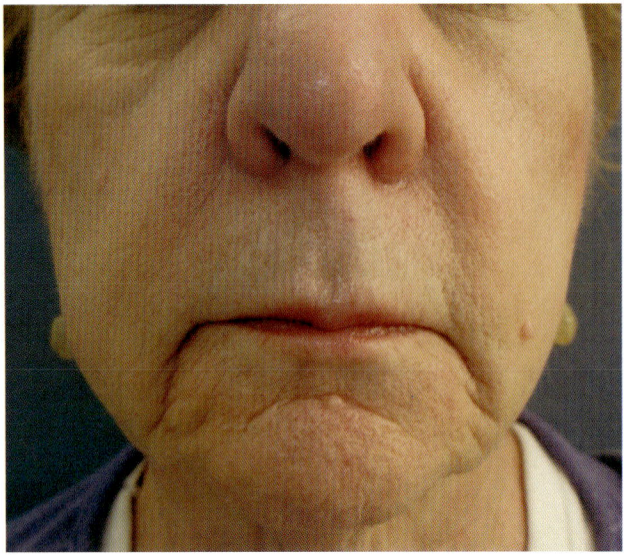

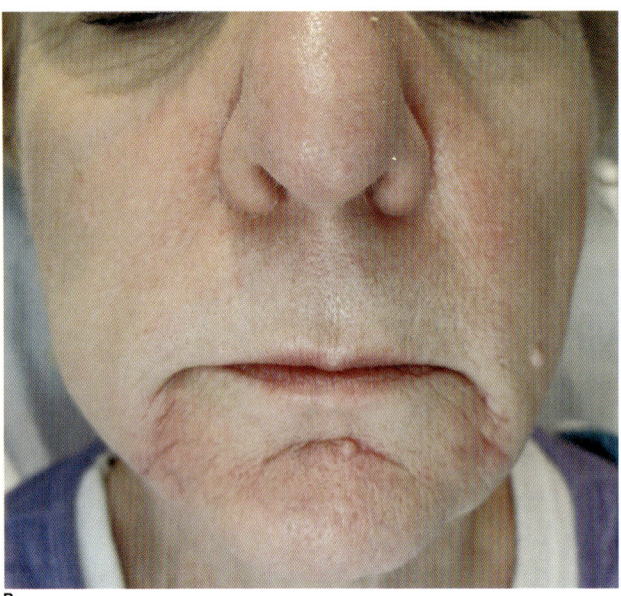

FIG. 6.7. *(A,B) Patient before injection into the marionette lines and four weeks posttreatment.*

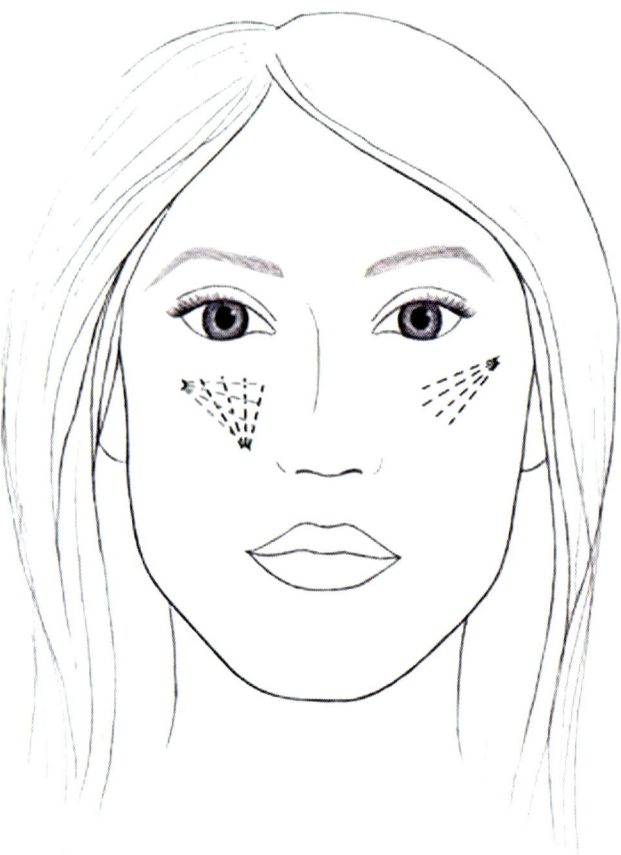

FIG. 6.8. *Threading and cross-hatching for treatment of the malar/submalar area. (Illustration courtesy of BioForm Medical, Inc.)*

(Figure 6.8). Care should be taken not to inject Radiesse above the infraorbital rim.

For best aesthetic results when using long-term fillers, the entire malar area should be augmented, not merely the areas where soft tissue deficiency is most obvious. This treatment of the region, rather than the specific defect, appears to signal a new direction in the use of soft tissue fillers. Many dermatologists began with correction of a line, for example, an NLF. Over time, dermatologists have begun to expand the scope of their treatment protocols, using regional volume enhancement as the treatment objective, rather than treatment of the defect in isolation.

For a smoother look and more natural feel, filler should be placed at the junction of the deep dermis and the subcutaneous tissue. For large volume augmentation, both the subcutaneous and the subdermal planes may be injected. Deeper implantation gives a more natural feel and allows larger volumes of material to be safely implanted.

HIV-Associated Facial Lipoatrophy

HIV-associated lipoatrophy is believed to be associated with metabolic disturbances in glucose and lipid metabolism related to the use of antiretroviral therapy, leading to changes in body composition. Although not life threatening, facial lipoatrophy may be very pronounced and obvious and may be associated with significant social stigma.[7] Though HIV-associated lipoatrophy cannot be "cured," it can be effectively treated with soft tissue fillers. Because of its innate biocompatibility and its volumizing properties, Radiesse is particularly well suited for augmentation of the submalar area in patients with HIV-associated lipoatrophy. When used for this purpose, larger volumes are required than typically used for the NLFs. Because of the large area treated, the material is typically injected using a cross-hatching, layered technique (Figure 6.9).

In a pivotal study of CaHA in patients with HIV-associated lipoatrophy, patient satisfaction was rated at 97–100 percent at every evaluation over an eighteen-month period. Subjective improvements in appearance were accompanied by increased skin thickness measurements.[7]

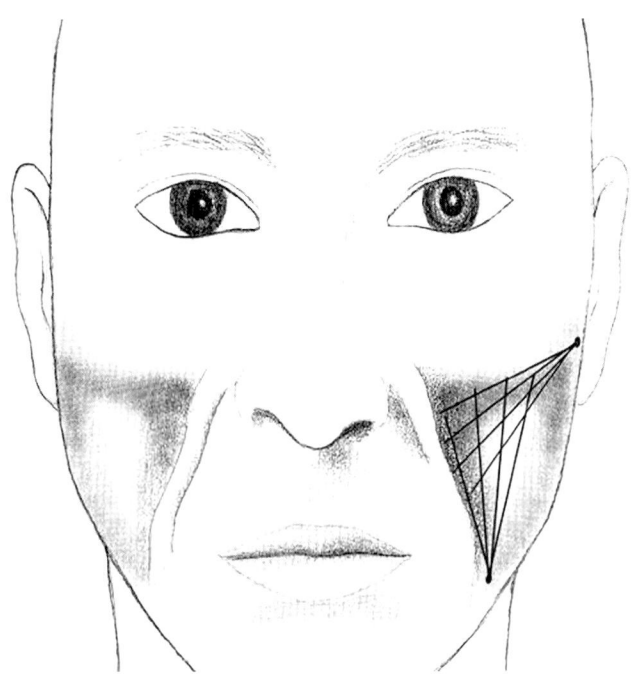

FIG. 6.9. *Treatment areas for individual with lipoatrophy. (Illustration courtesy of BioForm Medical, Inc.)*

POSTINJECTION CARE

Immediately after injection, the site should be gently massaged and molded by the treating physician to help ensure a smoother implant. Patients should not manipulate the treated area. Posttreatment care involves application of ice over the injection areas to reduce and limit tissue edema and ecchymosis. Patient follow-up visits are typically scheduled twelve weeks or later to provide refining treatments as necessary. Posttreatment photographs should be taken as soon as the injections have been completed and the washable markings removed.

POTENTIAL COMPLICATIONS

Radiesse enjoys an excellent safety profile with adverse events reported typical of that observed with other short-acting fillers such as collagen and hyaluronic acid. Patients may experience mild pain, erythema, and possible ecchymoses immediately after treatment. These effects should resolve within two weeks. The risk of ecchymosis and erythema can be minimized by having the patient discontinue all potential blood-thinning agents for two weeks before treatment, including aspirin and NSAIDs.[12] Further minimizing of bruising and swelling can be accomplished by taking time to inject the material slowly and gently into the tissues. Some physicians have found prophylactic administration of bromelain and arnica montana helpful for reducing severity of bruising.

As with any filler, CaHA should not be injected in the presence of foreign body reaction, inflammation, or infection.[1] Patients with a known predilection to herpesvirus infections of the lips should receive acyclovir or another oral antiviral agent prior to the use of CaHA in the perioral region.

The potential for serious adverse reactions with Radiesse appears to be low. There is no evidence of granuloma formation occurring with CaHA.

Although the presence of nodules visible through the skin has been reported, these nodules are technique related due to too superficial injection of CaHA or inappropriate use of CaHA. If such nodules occur, they can be easily reduced using aggressive massage techniques. It is rare that intralesional steroids or excision is required to remove accumulations of CaHA material.

CONCLUSIONS

Radiesse continues to demonstrate its utility as a longer lasting filler with the ability to correct moderate-to-severe defects (e.g., NLFs) and provide volume augmentation in the face (e.g., facial lipoatrophy).

As clinical experience with Radiesse has become more widespread and is increasingly well documented in the medical literature, it is possible to address certain misconceptions about CaHA as a cosmetic filler material. As previously described, the injected CaHA microspheres form a scaffold for fibroblastic activity. New tissue growth at the injection site mimics the surrounding tissue; there is no evidence of osteogenesis when CaHA is injected into soft tissue.[2,17]

Another question that has emerged is whether CaHA, which is radiopaque, might confound or impede interpretation of X-rays. This question was examined in a radiographic study of patients who were treated with CaHA for HIV-associated facial lipoatrophy or correction of NLFs. This study found that there are no overt radiographic safety concerns with CaHA and that its appearance on computed tomographic (CT) scans is distinct from surrounding bony tissues and does not interfere with normal analysis.[19] Interestingly, this study also provided evidence that CaHA particles do not migrate and remain localized at the injection site.

Another area of confusion is the erroneous association of CaHA with the formation of granulomas. There is no evidence of inflammatory reactions to CaHA leading to the formation of granulomatous nodules.[9,12,17] The appearance of visible nodules of CaHA material, which is *not* a granulomatous process, has been reported with the use of CaHA in the lip mucosae. This outcome can be prevented by avoiding the use of Radiesse in the lips.[1]

It is anticipated that as clinicians increasingly gain familiarity with Radiesse, new aesthetic and corrective applications will continue to emerge, and its profile as a volumizing longer lasting filler will garner it a unique place among available fillers.

REFERENCES

1. Goldberg DJ. Calcium hydroxylapatite. In: *Fillers in Cosmetic Dermatology*. Abingdon, England: Informa UK Ltd.; 2007.
2. Hubbard W. *BioForm Implants: Biocompatibility*. Franksville, WI: Bioform Inc., 2003.
3. Tzikas TL. Evaluation of Radiance™ FN soft tissue filler for facial soft tissue augmentation. *Arch Facial Plast Surg*. 2004; **6**:234–239.
4. Hobar PC, Pantaloni M, Byrd HS. Porous hydroxylapatite granules for alloplastic enhancement of the facial region. *Clin Plast Surg*. 2000; **27**(4):557–569.
5. Mayer RD, Dmochowski RR, Appell RA, et al. Multicenter, prospective, randomized 52-week trial of calcium hydroxylapatite versus bovine dermal collagen for treatment of stress urinary incontinence. *Urology*. 2007; **69**:876–880.
6. Kershen RT, Dmochowski RR, Appell RA. Beyond collagen: injectable therapies for the treatment of female stress urinary incontinence in the new millennium. *Urol Clin North Am*. 2002; **29**:559–574.
7. Silvers SL, Eviatar JA, Echavez MI, et al. Prospective, open-label, 18-month trial of calcium hydroxylapatite (Radiesse) for facial soft-tissue augmentation in patients with human immunodeficiency virus-associated lipoatrophy: one-year durability. *Plast Reconstr Surg*. 2006; **118**(Suppl):34S–45S.
8. Smith S, Busso M, McClaren M, Bass L. A randomized, bilateral, prospective and multi-center comparison of calcium hydroxylapatite microspheres in gel versus human-based collagen for the correction of nasolabial folds. *Dermatol Surg*. 2007; **33**:S112–S121.

9. Felderman LI. Radiesse™ for facial rejuvenation. *Cosmet Dermatol.* 2005; **18**(22):823–826.

10. Flaharty P. Radiance FN for facial plastic soft tissue filling. *Facial Plast Surg.* 2004; **20**(2):165–169.

11. Kanchwala SK, Holloway L, Buck LP. Reliable soft tissue augmentation: a clinical comparison of injectable soft-tissue fillers for facial-volume augmentation. *Ann Plast Surg.* 2005; **33**:30–35.

12. Ahn MS. Calcium hydroxylapatite: Radiesse. *Facial Plast Surg Clin North Am.* 2007; **15**:85–90.

13. Jacovella PF, Peiretti CB, Cunille D, et al. Long-lasting results with hydroxylapatite (Radiesse) facial filler. *Plast Reconstr Surg.* 2006; **118**(Suppl):15S–21S.

14. Stupak HD, Mouthrop THM, Wheatley P, et al. Calcium hydroxylapatite gel (Radiesse) injection for the correction of postrhinoplasty contour deficiencies and asymmetries. *Arch Facial Plast Surg.* 2007; **9**:130–136.

15. Becker H. Nasal augmentation with calcium hydroxylapatite in a carrier-based gel. *Plast Reconstr Surg.* 2008; **121**:2142–2147.

16. Busso M, Karlsberg PL. Check augmentation and rejuvenation using injectable calcium hydroxylapatite (Radiesse®). *Cosmet Dermatol.* 2006; **19**(9):583–588.

17. Marmur ES, Phelps R, Goldberg DJ. Clinical, histologic, and electron microscopic findings after injection of a calcium hydroxylapatite filler. *J Cosmet Laser Ther.* 2004; **6**:223–226.

18. Alam M, Yoo SS. Technique for calcium hydroxylapatite injection for correction of nasolabial fold depressions. *J Am Acad Dermatol.* 2007; **56**:285–289.

19. Carruthers A, Liebeskind B, Carruthers J, Forster BB. Radiographic and computed tomographic studies of calcium hydroxylapatite for treatment of HIV-associated facial lipoatrophy and correction of nasolabial folds. *Dermatol Surg.* 2008; **34**:S78–S84.

20. Hubbard W. *BioForm Implants: Durability.* Franksville, WI: Bioform Inc., 2002. Available at: http://www.radiesse.com/pdf/Durability.pdf. Accessed on June 10, 2007.

21. Jansen DA, Graivier MH. Evaluation of a calcium hydroxylapatite-based implant (Radiesse) for facial soft tissue augmentation. *Plast Reconstr Surg.* 2006; **118**(Suppl):22S–30S.

22. Moers-Carpi M, Tufet JO. Calcium hydroxylapatite versus nonanimal stabilized hyaluronic acid for the correction of nasolabial folds: a 12-month, multi-center, prospective, randomized, controlled split-face trial. *Dermatol Surg.* 2008; **34**:210–215.

23. Moers-Carpi M, Vogt S, Martinez Santos B, Planas J, Rovira Vallve S. A multi-center, randomized trial comparing Radiesse to Juvederm and Perlane for the treatment of nasolabial folds. *Poster presentation, annual meeting of Eur Acad of Derm and Venereology.* May 16–20, 2007; Vienna, Austria.

Chapter 7

ARTEFILL

by

Steven R. Cohen, MD, FACS and
Mark G. Rubin, MD

INTRODUCTION

The demand for safe, effective, long-lasting, and biocompatible dermal filler materials is increasing as a growing number of patients seek minimally invasive options for aesthetic improvement. For a substance or device to be amenable for soft tissue augmentation, in addition to producing the desired cosmetic results, the product must be well tolerated, exhibit a minimum of undesirable reactions, and be nonteratogenic, noncarcinogenic, and nonmigratory.[1] In addition, the material or device must be easy to use and provide predictable, persistent correction through reproducible implantation techniques. Finally, in the United States, the Food and Drug Administration (FDA) review and approval of such products not only substantiates they meet safety and efficacy requirements but also assures adherence to important manufacturing and product labeling requirements postapproval.

Numerous attempts have been made to develop safe biological (e.g., collagen, hyaluronic acid) or synthetic (man-made) materials to fill unwanted wrinkles and scars.[1,2] Currently, in the United States, there are about twelve or more different soft tissue fillers approved for cosmetic use; in Europe, there are approximately eighty CE marked approved cosmetic fillers with many more available worldwide. Historically, biologic filler materials that use "natural-based" core substances such as collagen and hyaluronic acid materials have predominated the marketplace. These materials, whether they are derived from a bioengineered or extracted from a natural source, typically have been modified to improve tolerability (e.g., removal of impurities) and modified to improve durability (e.g., cross-linked). Nonetheless, these products typically last no more than a year and therefore require repeat therapy over time to preserve.[3–6]

For patients who understand the risks and benefits of soft tissue therapy, there clearly is a role for products with greater persistence. No material can produce permanent correction given the aging dynamic of the skin, which continues to change over time; however, having a safe, effective, and more "semipermanent" or longer lasting soft tissue filler solution would offer some distinct advantages. Given the more liberal approval requirements in countries outside of the United States, more permanent nonresorbable soft tissue filler materials have been available for years. These products are typically based on synthetic man-made materials, and their quality has been variable.

Unfortunately, these products have been plagued by challenges with tolerability and have therefore developed a reputation of concern among the medical community.[7]

Intuitively, the requirements for such products need to be more rigorous given their "permanent" qualities. In retrospect, it has become clear that many of these products were commercialized before their time. Nonetheless, these experiences have driven home the essential requirements of biocompatibility, particle characteristics, purity, and the need for strict manufacturing requirements both precommercialization and postcommercialization for these more permanent nonresorbable filler materials.

In 2007, the first nonresorbable filler material, ArteFill (Artes Medical, San Diego, CA), was approved by the FDA in the United States. ArteFill is a novel polymethylmethacrylate (PMMA)-based filler material for the correction of nasolabial folds. The product is composed of nonresorbable PMMA microspheres, suspended in a water-based carrier gel composed of 3.5 percent purified bovine collagen, 92.6 percent buffered, isotonic water for injection, 0.3 percent lidocaine hydrochloride, 2.7 percent phosphate buffer, and 0.9 percent sodium chloride.[8] ArteFill is distinguished from all previous PMMA fillers in that its safety and efficacy have been demonstrated in well-controlled multicenter trials in approximately 391 subjects.[8] These original studies have been further supported by five-year follow-up evaluations in about 142 subjects.[9] The product is also distinguished by the inclusion of lidocaine to ease the discomfort associated with implant placement. This chapter reviews the history of PMMA technology as a filler material and the unique qualities and characteristics of ArteFill that distinguish it from other PMMA fillers that have emerged before it.

HISTORY OF PMMA AS A SOFT TISSUE FILLER

PMMA was first synthesized by the German chemist O. Rohm in 1902. This novel polymer was subsequently patented in 1928 by Rohm and Haas Company and has since been used in dentures, in prosthetic devices, in intraocular lenses, as a carrier for antibiotics, in pacemakers, and as bone cement in orthopedics and neurosurgery.[10] PMMA-based material has been studied as a potential soft tissue augmentation product since the early 1980s.[11]

The goal was to develop an augmentation material that would provide longer lasting augmentation. Nonresorbable biocompatible materials often stimulate collagen deposition – a reaction that may persist over a long period of time.[12] The search for the appropriate material led to PMMA given its success as a well-tolerated biomaterial.[13] The novel application as a soft tissue filler, however, required the material to be used in a different form. The use of the material as microspheres was consistent with the requirement of the final product being developed in an injectable dosage form. Theoretically, this approach would also allow the creation of a new collagen matrix around the network of microspheres after placement of the implant, potentially resulting in a longer term correction.

With this approach in mind, the first critical step in developing PMMA for soft tissue augmentation was to isolate microspheres large enough to avoid phagocytosis but small enough to allow injection into the deep dermis through a twenty-six-gauge needle by a technique called suspension polymerization.[14] Particle characteristics of implant materials, such as size and morphology, have long been known to be important for the biocompatibility and performance of soft tissue filler materials.[15] The literature demonstrates that microsphere-containing products have different safety and efficacy profiles based on the composition, morphology, and surface characteristics of the microspheres they contain.[16]

A first-generation product used in humans was called Arteplast.[13] The original suspension consisted of PMMA microspheres, 30–42 μm in diameter suspended in a gelatin-based carrier. This product was manufactured and clinically tested in Frankfurt, Germany, between 1989 and 1994.[17] Unfortunately, the PMMA microspheres in Arteplast had many small surface impurities that are believed to have caused an unacceptable rate of late foreign body granulomas. Of 578 subjects who received this product, 15 developed granulomas within six to eighteen months of injection.[18] These surface impurities adhered to the spheres as a result of electrostatic forces and resisted washing and sieve filtration. The limitation of producing microspheres with consistent particle size and limited impurities has been a shortcoming with the early stage of PMMA technology development.

In 1994, new purification and washing techniques were introduced. The sieving process was changed from a nylon fabric mesh to a metal mesh, and a complex washing and ultrasound procedure was devised that removed nanoparticles and electrical surface charges, which were thought to be the cause of foreign body reactions and granuloma formation. Another change made at the same time was the use of collagen as a carrier to replace the gelatin carrier, which is resorbed too quickly and thereby permits clumping of particles. The improved second-generation product, named Artecoll, was manufactured and distributed by Rofil Medical International B.V. in Breda, the Netherlands, as an injectable augmenting agent.[11] It is a suspension of 20 percent PMMA microspheres in an 80 percent bovine collagen solution as a delivery vehicle. This product has been used in Europe since approximately 1993 and in Canada since 1998.[11] Adverse responses observed

with injected Artecoll are early lump formation, which is fairly common, and later granuloma formation, which is uncommon, but the incidence is not well quantified. Small lumps, thought to be a technique-related issue due to the local collection of excess material, may occur for a period of time following Artecoll injection, particularly with too superficial placement or in certain anatomic locations such as the lips.[19] Fortunately, these other granulomatous changes though rare have been shown to improve over time with local therapy such as intralesional steroid therapy.[20,21]

Artecoll reportedly has been used worldwide (except in the United States and Japan) in more than 400,000 subjects.[22] This second generation of PMMA technology clearly benefited from the improved particle characteristics as compared to its predecessor, Arteplast. Examples of Artecoll PMMA particle characteristics using scanning electron microscopy (SEM) have recently been published by Piacquadio et al.[23] Of note, these authors demonstrated differences between the Artecoll products originating from Europe (ca. 2001) versus Canada (ca. 2005). The European version of Artecoll (see Figure 7.1A,B) has PMMA microspheres 32–40 μm in diameter with variable particle sizes and the presence of nanoparticles on the surface of microspheres. There were also some 20- and 5-μm particles noted with some sediment. The Artecoll product originating from Canada (see Figure 7.2A,B) has microspheres 30–50 μm in diameter, with negligible small sizes. The microspheres were observed to be smooth surfaced with slight surface irregularity and scant if any sediment. However, there were still some surface irregularities present that may have led to increased granuloma formation.

The European Union (CE Mark) has historically had less stringent requirements compared to the United States with respect to the approval of soft

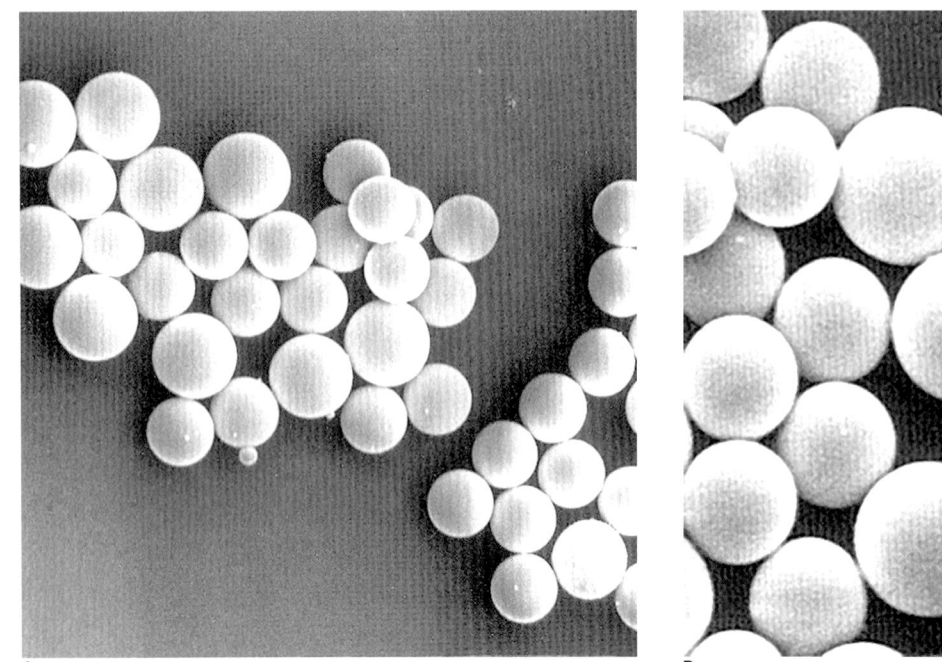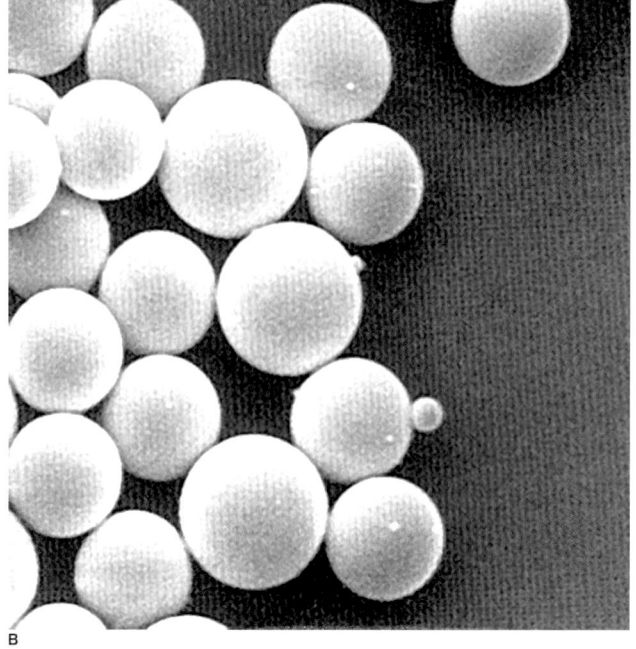

A

B

FIG. 7.1.   (A,B) SEM images of PMMA in Artecoll from Europe, approximately 2001 (reprinted with permission from Piacquadio, Smith, and Anderson, 2008).

tissue filler products. In the European Union, clinical validation of safety and efficacy of a new soft tissue filler material can be obtained from smaller human studies and/or by using supportive arguments based on referencing clinical data for other related products in the public domain. Consistent with this, there were no formal clinical research studies of a material nature to approve Artecoll or Arteplast.

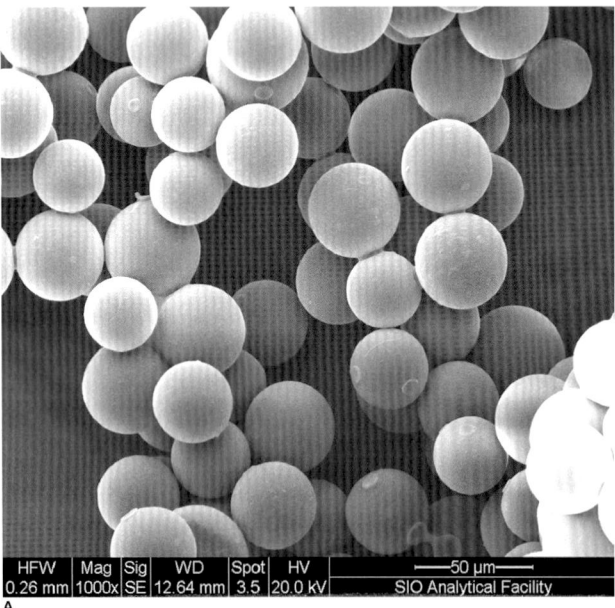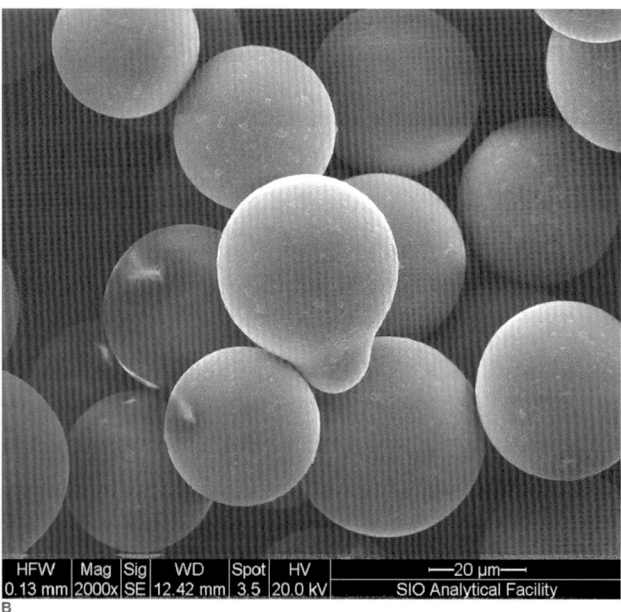

| HFW | Mag | Sig | WD | Spot | HV | ——50 µm—— |
| 0.26 mm | 1000x | SE | 12.64 mm | 3.5 | 20.0 kV | SIO Analytical Facility |

A

| HFW | Mag | Sig | WD | Spot | HV | ——20 µm—— |
| 0.13 mm | 2000x | SE | 12.42 mm | 3.5 | 20.0 kV | SIO Analytical Facility |

B

FIG. 7.2.   (A,B) SEM images of PMMA in Artecoll from Canada, year 2005 (reprinted with permission from Piacquadio, Smith, and Anderson, 2008).

Of equal importance, although the SEM analysis mentioned earlier implies continued improvement in the Artecoll particle characteristics (2001 vs. 2005), it clearly provides evidence to suggest that the PMMA products used outside the United States for the past two decades likely represent a continuum of products. It is not uncommon for clinicians to have a common view of a product such as Artecoll when in reality the product may have had multiple forms over time with potentially different therapeutic features with respect to safety and efficacy. To further complicate matters, detailed specifics about such manufacturing changes are typically not publicly disclosed.

In summary, these types of product dynamics make it virtually impossible to establish a therapeutic index (the balance between its safety and efficacy qualities) of a product that has likely continued to evolve over time. Given the early problems with PMMA-based fillers, it is particularly difficult for both patients and clinicians to have a clear understanding of this technology. However, the recent introduction of the first US FDA–approved PMMA soft tissue filler, substantiated by a large body of clinical data, has provided a basis to understand the risks and benefits of this technology for the first time. Moreover, since the second-generation product, Artecoll, was used in the pivotal FDA study, the highly controlled study yielded valuable information on the frequency of adverse events up to nearly five and one-half years after injection.[9]

ArteFill is a third-generation PMMA-based filler product that contains an optimized collagen matrix with microspheres that have enhanced uniformity and consistency as well as near elimination of nanoparticles (see Figure 7.3A,B) compared to the second-generation PMMA product and the original formulation, Arteplast. ArteFill was approved by the FDA in October 2006 for the correction of nasolabial folds, based on results of a US pivotal trial with the second-generation predecessor product, Artecoll. Since the initiation of the pivotal trial, substantial improvements in the second-generation PMMA product have been made in cooperation

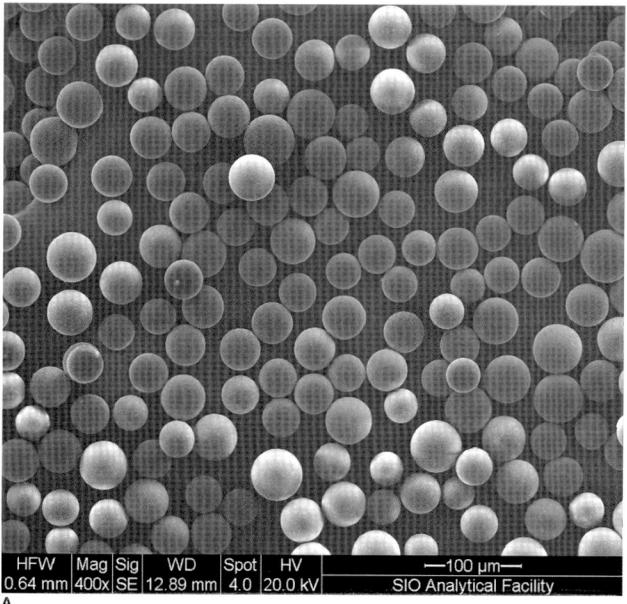
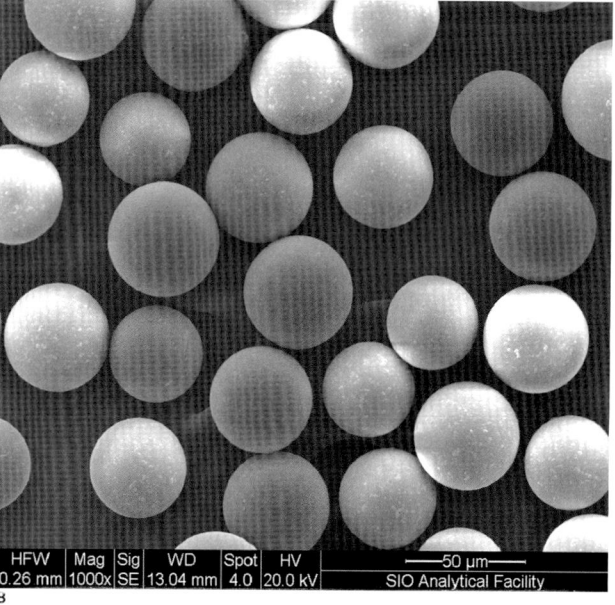

FIG. 7.3. (A,B) SEM images of PMMA in ArteFill from the United States, year 2007 (reprinted with permission from Piacquadio, Smith, and Anderson, 2008).

with the FDA, which are believed to have further improved the tolerability of the implant material. These additional refinements focused on further enhancement to the uniformity of PMMA particle characteristics, virtually eliminating particles less than 20 μm in size. Research suggests that particles less than 20 μm are easily phagocytized, which increases the chance of immunologic reactions.[24] Furthermore, the product is now manufactured in the United States using a more refined carrier matrix having bovine collagen that is sourced from a restricted closed herd in the United States. ArteFill is the only PMMA-based injectable product that has been approved by the FDA for the treatment of facial wrinkles.

SAFETY AND EFFICACY – PIVOTAL STUDY

ArteFill is the first PMMA filler that has been studied in well-controlled multicenter trials. As described before, the pivotal study used to support the approval of ArteFill was actually performed with the most recent version of Artecoll before the product underwent additional manufacturing improvements with respect to the collagen matrix and PMMA microspheres; however, for clarity in this chapter, the product is referred always as ArteFill consistent with the product's package insert.

The pivotal trial was a multicenter, randomized, double-blinded, controlled study intended to evaluate the safety and effectiveness of ArteFill compared to a collagen control (Zyplast; Inamed Corporation, Santa Barbara, CA) when used for cosmetic correction of contour deformities of the dermis of the face (data on file at Artes Medical). The study involved 251 men ($n = 22$) and women ($n = 229$) between the ages of twenty-eight and eighty-two at eight US centers; these participants received ArteFill or collagen as a control in 420 nasolabial folds, in addition to other facial wrinkles (glabella, radial upper lip lines, and corners of the mouth). One hundred twenty-eight subjects received ArteFill (108 were treated in the nasolabial fold), and 123 received collagen (104 treated in the nasolabial fold). Treatment effectiveness and safety were assessed at one, three, and six months after completion of the treatment course. In addition, long-term safety assessment was done with subjects randomized to the ArteFill treatment group twelve months after completion of the treatment course. Assessment of safety was based on the incidence of adverse events that were characterized by the severity and relation to the implant product.

Efficacy was determined using the Facial Fold Assessment (FFA) Scale.[25] The FFA Scale is a validated six-point, photometric index of the severity of nasolabial folds with the following classifications: 0 (no folds), 1 (folds just perceptible, about 0.1 mm), 2 (shallow folds, about 0.2 mm), 3 (moderately deep folds, about 0.5 mm), 4 (deep folds, most edges well defined, some redundant folds, about 1.0 mm), and 5 (very deep folds, about 2.0 mm). Standardized photographs were taken at designated evaluation time points during the trial. Independent, masked observers classified each nasolabial fold according to the FFA Scale. The mean score of three independent masked graders was designated as the primary efficacy measure. The primary efficacy endpoint was the improvement in masked observer FFA Scale ratings from pretreatment values to the six-month follow-up observation time point. As a secondary efficacy endpoint, investigators assessed the depth of the nasolabial folds using the same FFA Scale but observing the subjects in person rather than evaluating from photographs. Subjects receiving ArteFill demonstrated a significant nasolabial fold correction, superior to that of the collagen control at both three and six months postinjection based on masked observer and investigator FFA Scale ratings ($p < 0.001$; see Figures 7.4 and 7.5). The superiority of ArteFill was observed despite the fact that a substantially smaller quantity of material was used than in collagen

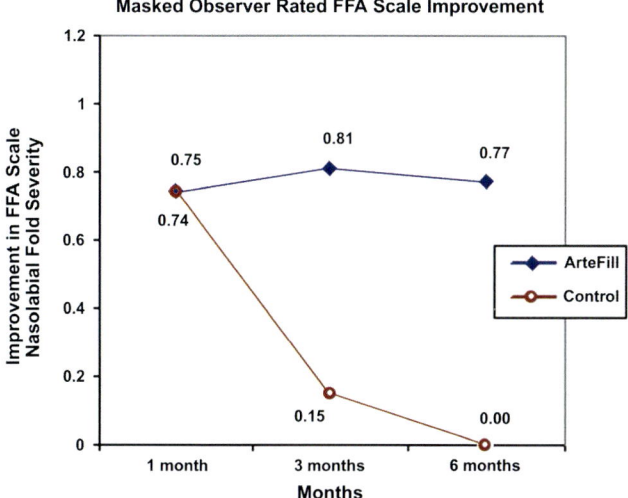

FIG. 7.4. *Comparison of mean improvement in masked observer FFA Scale ratings three and six months after ArteFill and control treatment.*

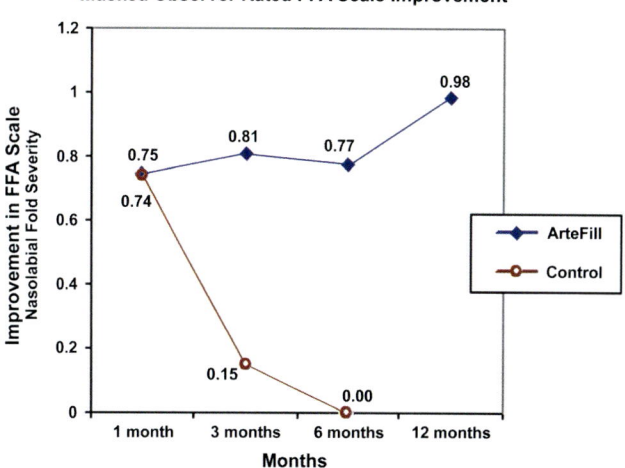

FIG. 7.6. *Greater nasolabial fold improvement for ArteFill at twelve months (M = 0.98) than for control at six months (M = 0.00) based on masked observer FFA Scale ratings (p < 0.001).*

control cases (0.82 vs. 1.46 cc per fold, $p < 0.001$). The effect of the collagen control treatment had returned to baseline by six months postinjection in contrast to the persistence demonstrated by ArteFill.

Efficacy data at twelve months (available for the ArteFill group only) demonstrated significant mean nasolabial fold correction relative to baseline (prior to any treatment) in masked observer and investigator FFA Scale ratings ($p < 0.001$). The nasolabial fold

area showed significantly greater improvement for ArteFill at twelve months ($M = 0.98$) than for control at six months ($M = 0.00$) based on masked observer FFA Scale ratings ($p < 0.001$). Similar results were found based on investigator FFA Scale ratings with greater nasolabial fold improvement for ArteFill at twelve months ($M = 2.07$) than for control at six months ($M = 0.01$; $p < 0.001$) (see Figures 7.6 and 7.7).

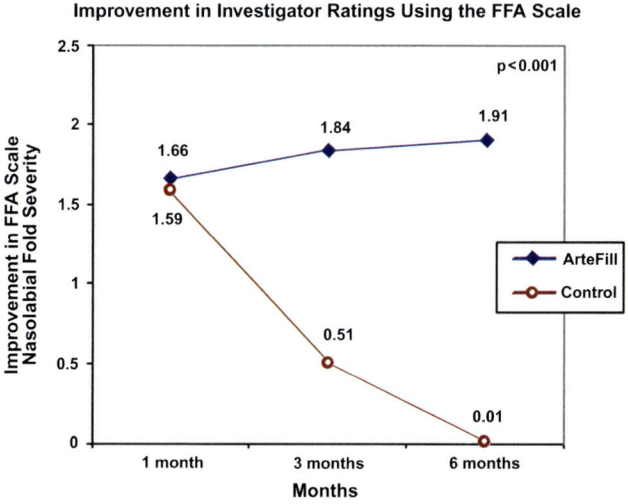

FIG. 7.5. *Comparison of mean improvement in investigator FFA Scale ratings three and six months after ArteFill and control treatment.*

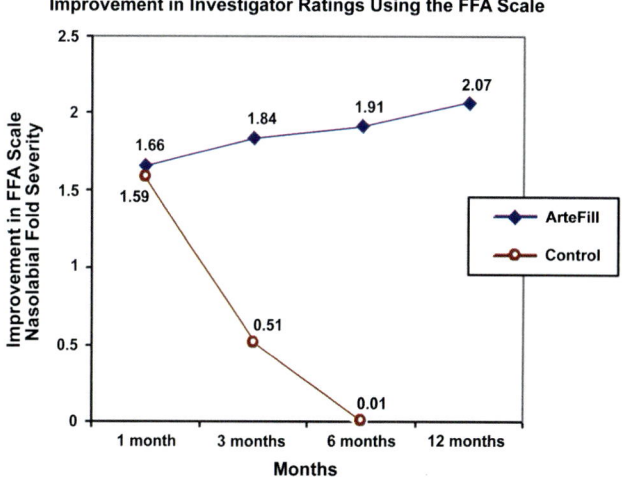

FIG. 7.7. *Greater nasolabial fold improvement for ArteFill at twelve months (M = 2.07) than for control at six months (M = 0.01) based on investigator FFA Scale ratings (p < 0.001).*

Secondary measures in this study included the investigator's assessment of success and the subject's assessment of satisfaction, both characterized using a nonparametric five-point scale, measured at one, three, and six months posttreatment (and twelve months for ArteFill subjects). Investigator rating of success was done using the following five-point rating scale: 1 = completely successful, 2 = very successful, 3 = moderately successful, 4 = somewhat successful, and 5 = not at all successful. Subject satisfaction was done using the following five-point rating scale: 1 = very satisfied, 2 = satisfied, 3 = somewhat satisfied, 4 = dissatisfied, and 5 = very dissatisfied. Descriptive statistics were used to characterize the investigator ratings of success and the subject's assessment of satisfaction with nasolabial fold treatment. The means are illustrated in Figures 7.8

and 7.9. By month 3, significantly more successful investigator ratings were obtained for ArteFill ($M = 1.90$) than for control ($M = 3.07$; $p < 0.001$). The significant difference in investigator ratings of success between ArteFill ($M = 1.73$) and control ($M = 4.05$) appeared more pronounced by month 6 ($p < 0.001$). Mean investigator success ratings of ArteFill were roughly at the "very successful" level at all follow-up points. Similar to the investigator ratings of success, more satisfactory subject ratings were obtained for ArteFill ($M = 2.16$) than for control ($M = 2.78$) by month 3 ($p = 0.001$). Again, the difference in subject satisfaction between ArteFill ($M = 2.02$) and control ($M = 3.52$) was more pronounced by month 6 ($p < 0.001$). Mean subject satisfaction ratings were generally at the "satisfied" level at all follow-up points.

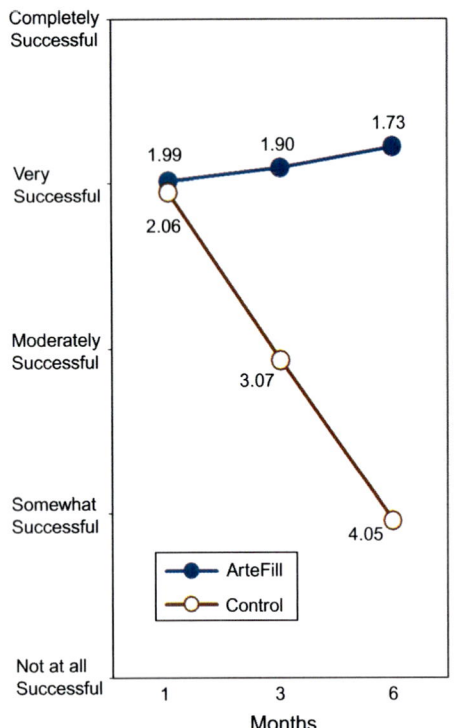

FIG. 7.8. *Mean investigator success ratings of the nasolabial fold area at one, three, and six months after treatment with ArteFill and control.*

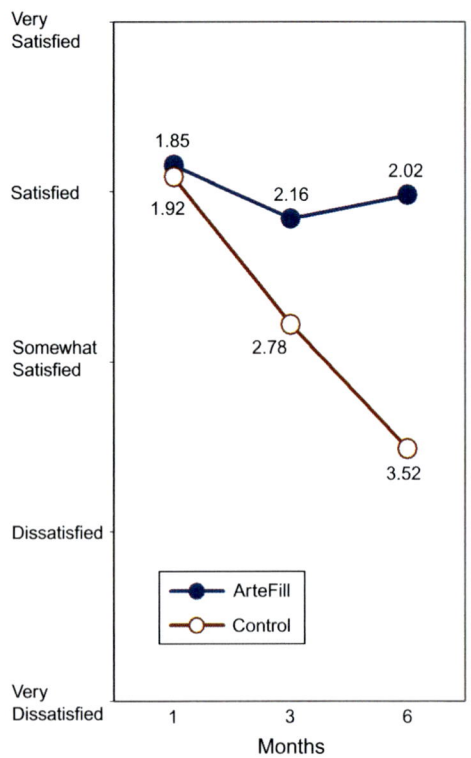

FIG. 7.9. *Mean subject ratings of satisfaction of the nasolabial fold area at one, three, and six months after treatment with ArteFill and control.*

Of the 251 subjects treated, 37 experienced a total of sixty-two adverse events. No subject experienced a serious unanticipated adverse device effect. ArteFill had a somewhat more favorable adverse event profile than the collagen control in this study but not materially different. Twenty-six adverse events were reported in twenty subjects in the ArteFill group in comparison to the thirty-six events reported in sixteen subjects in the collagen control group. Of these reported adverse events, five adverse events were determined as being unrelated to the implant material by the investigator (two for ArteFill, three for collagen control). In addition, the events are classified as mild, moderate, or severe as determined by the investigator. Finally, an additional classification was assigned if the implant was removed or the area was drained. In the case of ArteFill, one such case was reported, and it was related to mild lumpiness, which on biopsy was noted to be "actinic keratosis versus verrucous keratosis." In the case of the collagen control, two such cases were reported, both of which were severe local abscesses deemed as definitely related to the treatment by the investigator. A summary list of adverse events is shown in Table 7.1.

TABLE 7.1. Reported Adverse Events from ArteFill and Control Collagen Injections for the Twelve-Month Pivotal Study

	Number of Events							
	ArteFill				Control			
	Severity of Event, as Determined by Investigator			Removal or Drainage[a]	Severity of Event, as Determined by Investigator			Removal or Drainage[a]
Event	Mild	Moderate	Severe		Mild	Moderate	Severe	
Lumpiness at injection area more than 1 month after injection	6(1[b]) (1[c])	2	0	1[d](mild)	1	1	2	
Persistent swelling or redness	5	2	0		9(1[c])	3	1	
Increased sensitivity	4	0	0		0	0	1	
Rash, itching more than 48 hours after injection	2	0	0		0	2	0	
Blurred vision	0	1	0		0	0	0	
Flu-like symptoms	0	1	0		1[c]	0	0	
Recurrence of existing herpes labialis	1	0	0		0	0	0	
Sensitization reactions	0	0	0		2	3	1	
Abscess	0	0	0		0	1	2	2 (severe)
Visibility of puncture area	0	0	0		0	2	0	
Granuloma or enlargement of the implant	0	0	0		0	0	1	
Infection	0	0	0		0	0	1	
Other local complications	1	0	0		1[c]	0	0	
Other systemic complications	0	1[c]	0		0	0	0	
Severe illness, trauma, death	0	0	0		0	0	1[c]	
Total adverse events	19	7	0	1	14	12	10	2
	26				36			
Total subjects with adverse events	21			1	16			2
Total subjects treated	128				123			
Percent of subjects with adverse events	16.4			0.8	13.0			1.6

[a]Adverse events with removal or drainage are included in mild/moderate/severe counts.
[b]Using contrary to protocol (lip augmentation).
[c]Not related to implant.
[d]Pathology showed no foreign body reaction. Diagnosis of seborrheic keratosis. Not related to implant.

SAFETY AND EFFICACY: FIVE-YEAR FOLLOW-UP STUDY

To further substantiate the durability of ArteFill, a long-term five-year follow-up safety and efficacy study based on subjects enrolled in the original US multicenter pivotal study was performed.[9] The same methodology used in the pivotal study to substantiate the safety and efficacy of ArteFill was applied to evaluate subjects five years after their last treatment. The primary objective of the study was to determine efficacy for nasolabial folds based on masked observers' FFA Scale evaluations and safety using unanticipated event assessments. Secondary objectives were to evaluate efficacy by means of investigators' FFA Scale evaluations, investigators' success ratings, subjects' satisfaction ratings, and masked observers' FFA Scale evaluations for five years versus six months.

All of the investigators (eight US sites) involved in the original pivotal trial participated in the five-year follow-up study. The study included subjects initially randomized to be treated with ArteFill ($n = 128$) plus subjects in the collagen control group that elected to crossover to ArteFill treatment at the conclusion of their six-month collagen control treatment period ($n = 106$), for a total of 234 potential subjects. On or about the five-year anniversary date from their last treatment, each investigator contacted his or her ArteFill subject(s) by telephone and/or certified letter and encouraged them to enroll in the trial. From the original pivotal trial, 145 subjects (145/234 or 62 percent) responded to queries to participate in the study. Three subjects, however, were excluded from the efficacy analysis because their long-term follow-up period was less than 4.5 years. Of the remaining 142 subjects, there were 15 males and 127 females (mean age = 52.4 years); 82 subjects were from the original ArteFill group (64.1 percent) and 60 subjects in the

crossover group (56.6 percent), with a mean follow-up period of 5.36 years (range: 4.53–6.32 years) after their final treatment with ArteFill. Comparison of the original ArteFill and crossover groups revealed no significant difference in terms of follow-up rates (chi-square, $p = 0.245$). During the pivotal trial, ArteFill had been used to treat a variety of other anatomic sites (e.g., glabellar folds, mouth corners). In the five-year follow-up study, however, the focus was limited to the FDA-approved indication only, the treatment of nasolabial folds. In the group of five-year follow-up subjects, 124 had nasolabial fold corrections and provided the basis for the efficacy evaluation.

ArteFill maintained significant cosmetic correction in nasolabial folds five years after last treatment compared to baseline based on masked observer FFA Scale ratings ($n = 119$). Five of the 124 nasolabial fold subjects were excluded from analysis because they did not have either baseline or five-year photographs. Figure 7.10 shows an improvement of 1.01 points in masked observer FFA Scale ratings for this time period ($p < 0.001$). Similarly, there was an improvement of 1.67 points in investigator FFA Scale ratings ($n = 122$) for this time period as well ($p < 0.001$; see Figure 7.11). It is also interesting to note that there is continued improvement from the six-month to five-year time point based on the masked evaluator photographic scoring, a period during which no additional treatment was administered ($p < 0.002$). This change, however, was not seen based on live investigator assessments, but the degree of improvement noted by the investigator reflected approximately a 50 percent greater degree of wrinkle improvement (see comparison Figure 7.10 vs. Figure 7.11). This change is consistent with the proposed mechanism of action for this product where the PMMA microspheres are thought to induce persistent new collagen formation (see Figure 7.12). Actual results are

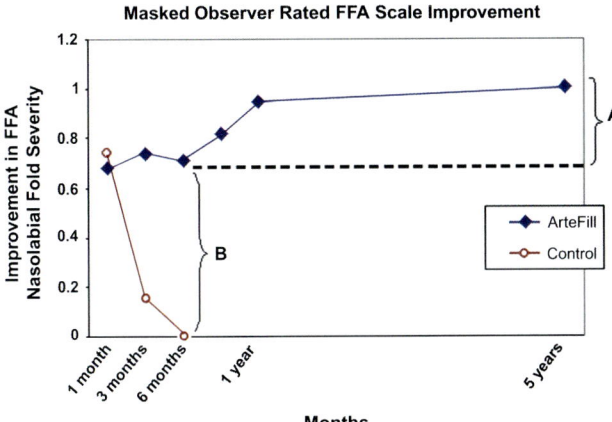

FIG. 7.10. *Mean improvement in masked observer FFA Scale ratings after ArteFill treatment over a period of five years. (A) Continuous improvement of ArteFill between six months (0.71) and five years (1.01; p < 0.002). (B) ArteFill (0.71) shows marked improvement over "collagen" control (0.00) at six months (p < 0.001).*

illustrated in photographs of a male (Figure 7.13) and female subject (Figure 7.14). These photographs, evaluated by three independent masked evaluators as done previously in the pivotal study, demonstrate improvement indicative of the mean FFA profile in Figure 7.10 over the five-year period.

Crossover subjects, those originally treated in the collagen control group that elected to have ArteFill

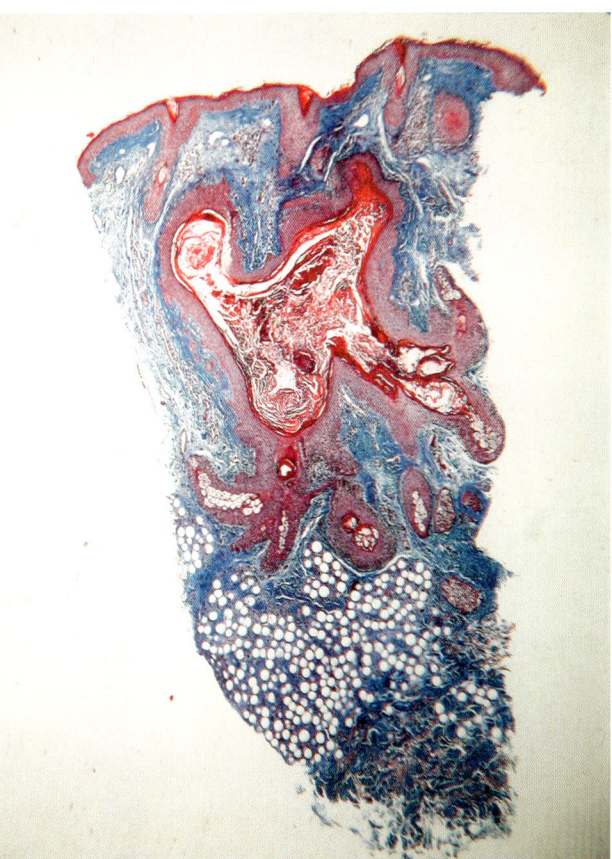

FIG. 7.12. *A biopsy of facial skin showing uniform vacuoles consistent with PMMA microspheres surrounded by deposited collagen twelve months after ArteFill implantation.*

treatment at six months, were evaluated as a subset. The results were significant for nasolabial folds ($p < 0.001$) with ArteFill showing significantly greater improvement after five years ($M = 0.91$) than the collagen-induced (control) improvement measured after six months ($M = 0.01$).

Secondary measures in this study included the investigator's assessment of success and the subject's assessment of satisfaction, both characterized using the same nonparametric five-point scale from the original pivotal trial. Consistent with the results obtained during the original pivotal study, both the investigator and the subject continued to have a very favorable impression of the therapy even five years

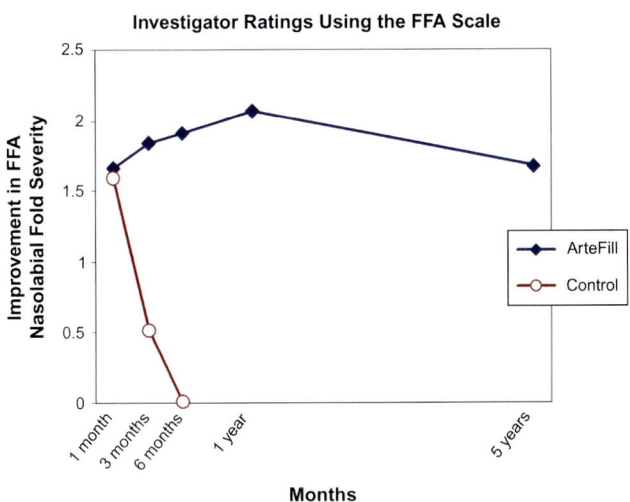

FIG. 7.11. *Mean improvement in investigator FFA Scale ratings after ArteFill treatment over a period of five years.*

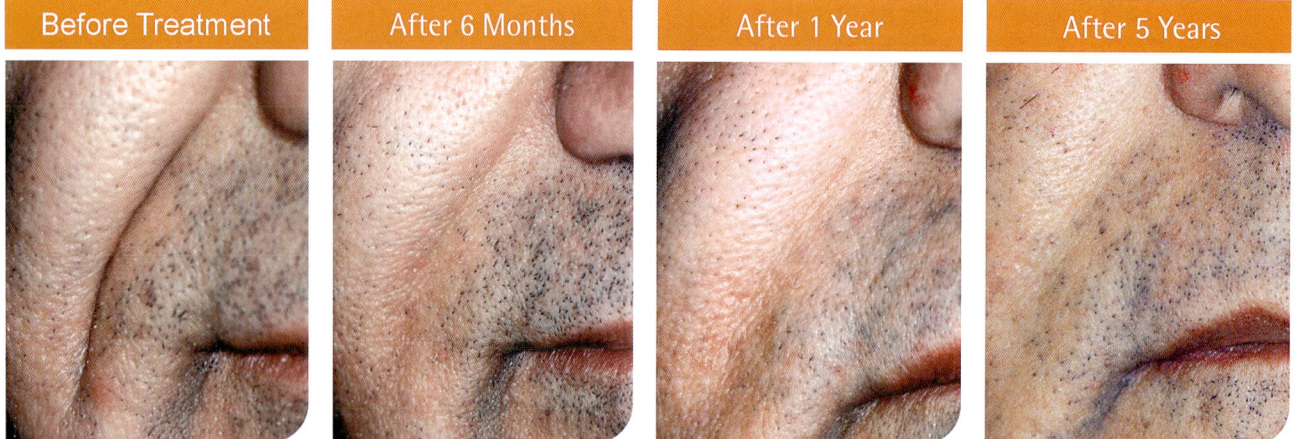

FIG. 7.13. *Before and after photographs of a male patient from baseline to year 5. This subject had no additional cosmetic procedures during the five-year follow-up period (reprinted with permission from Cohen et al., 2006).*

after their last treatment. As detailed in Figure 7.15, 90 percent of investigators described the cosmetic effect as "completely successful" or "very successful" (*N* = 123). Similarly, 90 percent of subjects described themselves as "very satisfied" or "satisfied" with the cosmetic outcome as illustrated in Figure 7.16.

In this five-year follow-up study, safety was evaluated in 145 subjects. There were twenty-eight total adverse events reported. Twenty treatment-related adverse events were distributed among fifteen subjects with one subject having three severe treatment–related adverse events. Four subjects had four severe

treatment–unrelated adverse events. A summary of adverse events that occurred since the last evaluation in the ArteFill pivotal trial is shown in Table 7.2. Mild treatment–related adverse events occurred in 8.3 percent of the total population; moderate treatment–related adverse events were reported in 1.4 percent and severe treatment–related adverse events in 0.7 percent. The most common treatment–related adverse event was lumpiness, 80 percent (8/10) of which was deemed mild.

Two subjects were assessed by the investigators as having "granuloma or enlargement of the implant." In one subject, a late-occurring (about five years

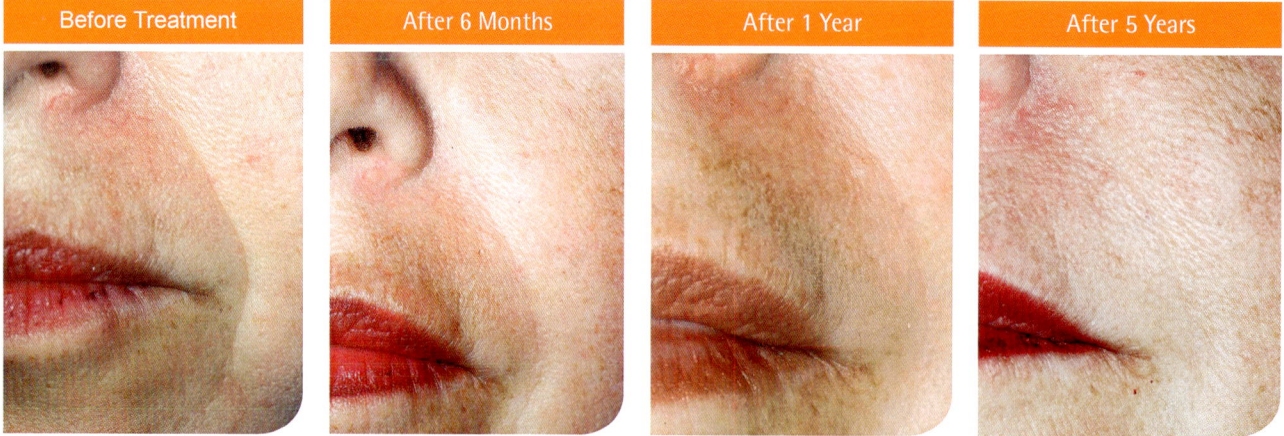

FIG. 7.14. *Before and after photographs of a female patient from baseline to year 5. This subject had no additional cosmetic procedures during the five-year follow-up period (reprinted with permission from Cohen et al., 2006).*

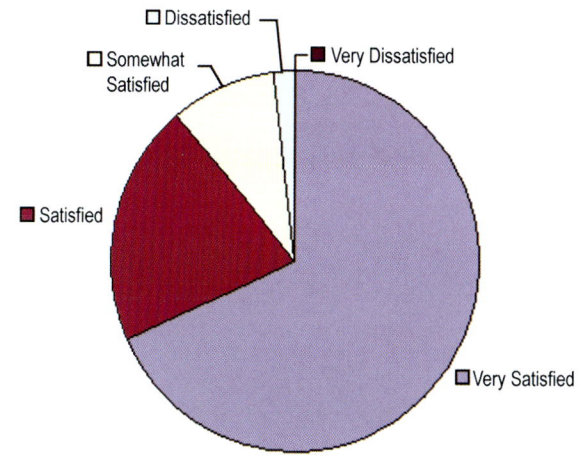

FIG. 7.15. Investigators' success ratings at five-year follow-up visit.

FIG. 7.16. Subjects' satisfaction ratings at five-year follow-up visit.

posttreatment) change in the nasolabial fold area was characterized by an inflammatory reaction with associated lumpiness. This event was rated as "severe" and was determined to be "definitely related" to the implant by the investigator. This adverse event essentially resolved other than minimal residual change with intralesional steroid therapy. In the second

subject, an early developing (about six months after the last treatment) lip and melolabial fold change was characterized by an inflammatory reaction with associated lumpiness. This event was rated as one of "moderate" severity and was determined to be "definitely related" to the implant by the investigator. The affected area was managed by an intraoral surgical

TABLE 7.2. ArteFill Five-Year Follow-Up Adverse Events Summary

	Related			Not Related			
	Mild	Moderate	Severe	Mild	Moderate	Severe	Unknown
Lumpiness	8	1	1				
Increased sensitivity	2						
Persistent swelling or redness	1		1				
Sensitization reaction	1	1					
Granuloma or enlargement of implant[a]		1	1				
Other – mild prominence of implant	1						
Other – occasional pain when scrubbing face	1						
Other – basal cell carcinoma					2		
Other – scaly area mid-right upper lip				1			
Systemic – breast cancer						3	
Systemic – death due to cardiac failure						1	
Systemic – Alzheimer's							1
Totals:	**14**	**3**	**3**	**1**	**2**	**4**	**1**
Number of subjects with adverse events	12	2	1	1[b](0)	2	4[c](3)	1
Percent of subjects with adverse events ($n = 145$)	8.3	1.4	0.7	0.7[b] (0)	1.4	2.8[c] (2.1)	0.7

[a]Clinical enlargement of implant, but no histologic confirmation of foreign body reaction.
[b]Subject also had a related adverse event.
[c]One subject also had a related adverse event.
Note: There were three subjects with events included in this table that did not attend a study visit for safety evaluation and are therefore not included in the $n = 145$.

excision in conjunction with intralesional steroid injections.

DISCUSSION

Typically, soft tissue implant materials are eventually broken down by the body and therefore require frequent repeat injections over time to maintain correction. The apparent key point of difference for ArteFill is the product's ability to promote and sustain the patient's own collagen production. This theory is supported by the histologic appearance of the implant material (Figure 7.12) that demonstrates a tight network of collagen around the PMMA microspheres in a fashion similar to that seen with microdroplet silicone.

The development history of PMMA as a soft tissue filler technology unfortunately started out somewhat encumbered and therefore has resulted in safety concerns given poor quality products introduced early on. With the advent of this third-generation PMMA technology, the technology now appears to have a good safety profile that is consistent with other soft tissue filler products in this category. Of greatest concern to clinicians has been complications related to granulomatous reactions seen with more permanent fillers. Fortunately, these reactions appear to be rare with ArteFill (actually none have been reported at the time of this chapter being written); however, their true incidence remains to be quantified. Of equal importance, most of these reactions seem to be responsive to therapy (e.g., intralesional corticosteroids). Nonetheless, more work still needs to be done to fully understand the true therapeutic index of this therapy. Consistent with that goal, a long-term study evaluating ArteFill was initiated in the first quarter of 2008. This study is a prospective, multicenter, open-label trial with 1,000 subjects designed to further characterize the safety profile of this novel technology over a period of five years. Currently, over 600 subjects have been enrolled into the treatment phase of the study, and no unanticipated adverse events have been reported to date.

Presently, ArteFill is the only nonresorbable soft tissue filler material approved by the FDA for the correction of nasolabial folds. The product is distinguished by its long-term durability with evidence of meaningful persistent correction exceeding five years posttreatment in some patients. Such results are unparalleled in comparison to other fillers currently available in the United States. This product, however, should not be viewed as a single treatment solution in that patients may need repeat treatment over time to maintain an optimized correction given the changing dynamic of the aging face or to supplement the correction they obtained with their initial treatment, be it with more ArteFill or other filler materials. Similarly, we do not believe this product is suitable for every patient. Given the high probability of persistence with ArteFill, this product is likely best suited for your "experienced" patients that are comfortable with the benefits of soft tissue therapy. It is also important that your patient understands that although the material itself has a persistent or nonresorbable component, future supplemental correction may be needed for the reasons outlined earlier, although far less so than with other soft tissue fillers. In summary, this novel technology possesses unique qualities that clearly distinguish it from all other filler materials. This product has carved out a definitive role in the soft tissue therapeutic armamentarium that will likely grow as both patients and physicians become more familiar with the technology.

REFERENCES

1. A.W. Klein and M.L Elson. The history of substances for soft tissue augmentation. *Dermatologic Surgery*, **26** (2000), 1096–1105.
2. C.A. Murray, D. Zloty and L. Warshawski. The evolution of soft tissue fillers in clinical practice. *Dermatology Clinics*, **23** (2005), 343–363.

3. P. Andre. Evaluation of the safety of a non-animal stabilized hyaluronic acid (NASHA – Q – Medical, Sweden) in European countries: a retrospective study from 1997 to 2001. *Journal of the European Academy of Dermatology and Venereology*, **18** (2004), 422–425.

4. J.T. Cheng, S.W. Perkins and M.M. Hamilton. Collagen and injectable fillers. *Otolaryngologic Clinics of North America*, **35** (2002), 73–85.

5. N.J. Lowe, C.A. Maxwell, P. Lowe, M.G. Duick and K. Shah. Hyaluronic acid skin fillers: adverse reactions and skin testing. *Journal of the American Academy of Dermatology*, **45** (2001), 930–933.

6. G.D. Monheit and K.M. Coleman. Hyaluronic acid fillers. *Dermatologic Therapy*, **19** (2006), 141–150.

7. P. Andre, N.J. Lowe, A. Parc, T.H. Clerici and U. Zimmermann. Adverse reactions to dermal fillers: a review of European experiences. *Journal of Cosmetic and Laser Therapy*, **7** (2005), 171–176.

8. ArteFill Instructions for Use. San Diego, CA, Artes Medical, Inc., 2006.

9. S.R. Cohen, C.F. Berner, M. Busso, M.C. Gleason, D. Hamilton, R.E. Holmes, J.J. Romano, P.R. Rullan, M.P. Thaler, Z. Ubogy and T.R. Vecchione. ArteFill: a long-lasting injectable wrinkle filler material-summary of the U.S. Food and Drug Administration trials and a progress report on 4- to 5-year outcomes. *Plastic and Reconstructive Surgery*, **118** (2006), 64S–76S.

10. G. Lemperle, N. Hazan-Gauthier and M. Lemperle. PMMA microspheres (Artecoll) for skin and soft-tissue augmentation. Part II: clinical investigations. *Plastic and Reconstructive Surgery*, **96** (1995), 627–634.

11. G. Lemperle, J.J. Romano and M. Busso. Soft tissue augmentation with Artecol: 10-year history, indications, techniques, and complications. *Dermatologic Surgery*, **29** (2003), 573–587.

12. M. Mattioli-Belmonte, G. Giavaresi, G. Biagini, L. Virgili, M. Giacomini, M. Fini, F. Giantomassi, D. Natali and P. Torricelli. Tailoring biomaterial compatibility: in vivo tissue response versus in vitro cell behavior. *International Journal of Artificial Organs*, **26** (2003), 1077–1085.

13. G. Lemperle, II. Ott, U. Charrier, J. Hecker and M. Lemperle. PMMA microspheres for intradermal implantation: Part I. Animal research. *Annals of Plastic Surgery*, **26** (1991), 57–63.

14. H.G. Yuan, G. Kalfas and W.H. Ray. Suspension polymerization. *Polymer Reviews*, **31** (1991), 215–299.

15. K. Laeschke. Biocompatibility of microparticles into soft tissue fillers. *Seminars in Cutaneous Medicine and Surgery*, **23** (2004), 214–217.

16. B.F. Matlaga, L.P. Yasenchak and T.N. Salthouse. Tissue response to implanted polymers: the significance of shapes. *Journal of Biomedical Materials Research*, **10** (1976), 391–397.

17. G. Lemperle, S. de Fazio and P. Nicolau. ArteFill: a third-generation permanent dermal filler and tissue stimulator. *Clinics in Plastic Surgery*, **33** (2006), 551–565.

18. G. Lemperle, R. Rietz and M. Lemperle. First clinical experiences with Arteplast: PMMA microspheres injected beneath wrinkles and dermal defects. In *Plastic Surgery*, **Vol. 2**, ed. U.T. Hinderer. (Amsterdam: Elsevier, 1992), pp. 539–541.

19. A. Carruthers and J.D.A. Carruthers. Polymethylmethacrylate microspheres/collagen as a tissue augmenting agent: personal experience over 5 years. *Dermatologic Surgery*, **31** (2005), 1561–1565.

20. J.S. Conejo-Mir, S.S. Guirado and M.A. Munoz. Adverse granulomatous reaction to Artecoll treated by intralesional 5-fluorouracil and triamcinolone injections. *Dermatologic Surgery*, **32** (2006), 1079–1082.

21. A. Gelfer, A. Carruthers, J. Carruthers, F. Jang and S.C. Bernstein. The natural history of polymethylmethacrylate microspheres granulomas. *Dermatologic Surgery*, **33** (2007), 614–620.

22. Artecoll Physician's Brochure. Breda, The Netherlands, Rofil Medical International B.V., 2005.

23. D. Piacquadio, S. Smith and R. Anderson. A comparison of commercially available polymethylmethacrylate-based soft tissue fillers. *Dermatologic Surgery*, **34** (2008), S48–S52.

24. G. Lemperle, V. Morehenn, V. Pestonjamasp and R.L. Gallo. Migration studies and histology of injectable microspheres of different sizes in mice. *Plastic and Reconstructive Surgery*, **113** (2004), 1380–1390.

25. G. Lemperle, R.E. Holmes, S.R. Cohen and S.M. Lemperle. A classification of facial wrinkles. *Plastic and Reconstructive Surgery*, **108** (2001), 1735–1750.

AUGMENTATION FILLERS IN COSMETIC DERMATOLOGY: SILICONE

by

Neil S. Sadick, MD, Chad Prather, MD, and Derek Jones, MD

INTRODUCTION

As the armamentarium of fillers for soft tissue augmentation expands, physicians and patients continue to seek those that approach criteria for the "ideal filler." Regardless of treatment area, the ideal filler would demonstrate versatility, biocompatibility, consistency of results, a natural feel, an excellent safety profile, and a superb cost-to-benefit ratio. Furthermore, it would be easy to inject, have minimal side effects, and not require allergy testing. The ideal filler would also achieve some degree of longevity and, arguably, permanence.

Liquid injectable silicone (LIS) is the original permanent, synthetic soft tissue–augmenting filler that may be employed for a variety of cutaneous and subcutaneous atrophies. Used worldwide for at least forty years, it distinctively meets a majority of the criteria that would define the ideal filler, including versatility, reliability of results, a natural feel, and an excellent cost-to-benefit ratio. When LIS is appropriately administered with the microdroplet serial puncture technique, patients may obtain enduring correction of scars, rhytids, and depressions, as well as lasting augmentation of lips and other facial contour atrophies and deformities.

However, the "permanence" of LIS refers to the enduring nature of the product in vivo rather than a "permanent" cosmetic result. Although the progressive tissue volume loss of aging will continue to occur, the degree of correction due to placement of LIS will persist. For this reason, silicone and other permanent fillers are much less forgiving than temporary fillers, in that overcorrection or undesired augmentation will also persist. Hence, experience and precise technique are prerequisites to favorable patient outcomes. Physicians should only use LIS after extensive training in the proper technique and in the appropriate patient. Candidates for treatment should have clear treatment objectives and sufficient insight into the goal of gradual augmentation over multiple treatment sessions. Patients who desire immediate correction or are uncertain of treatment aims are better treated with shorter duration, temporary fillers rather than with LIS.

BASIC SCIENCE

The broad term "silicone" encompasses a family of synthetic polymers based on elemental silicon (Si), a relatively inert element that is essential to humans in small amounts and accounts for over 25 percent of the earth's crust by mass. Polymers in the silicone family may exist in solid (elastomer), liquid, and gel states, with various chemical, physical, mechanical, and thermal properties. Synthetic polymers also vary with regard to purity, sterility, and biocompatibility. Although various silicone polymers are widely employed for medical use, polydimethylsiloxane is the LIS specifically used for soft tissue augmentation. The molecular structure of this colorless, odorless, nonvolatile oil consists of repeating dimethylsiloxane units with terminal trimethylsiloxane ends (Figure 8.1).

Viscosity is of practical importance when comparing the various liquid silicones. The viscosity of a given silicone oil is dependent on the chain length of dimethylsiloxane units. Longer chain molecules demonstrate a higher viscosity, and individual polymers are formulated to a set viscosity dependent on mean chain length. Silicone viscosity is expressed in centistokes (cs), with 1 cs equal to the viscosity of water. Practically, those LIS products employed for injection into the human body have a viscosity of 350 cs (similar to mineral oil), 1,000 cs (similar to honey), or 5,000 cs, and viscosity remains stable after tissue implantation.

LIS has not been found to be carcinogenic and has demonstrated "an enviable record of safety" according to a 1998 National Science Panel investigating its use.[1] Its mechanism of augmentation is twofold: It causes both the gross displacement of dermal and subcutaneous tissue and the eventuation of tissue fibroplasia, defined as the deposition of new collagen. After an initial localized inflammatory reaction consisting of neutrophil migration and limited macrophage phagocytic activity, fibroblasts deposit a thin-walled collagen capsule around the silicone microdroplet.[2] This capsule effectively anchors the microdroplet in place and prevents migration (Figure 8.2). Furthermore, pure LIS is not altered in vivo, although small amounts may be phagocytosed and enter the reticuloendothelial system.[3]

HISTORY AND CONTROVERSY

Soon after Dow Corning introduced the first commercially available silicone for industrial wartime use in the 1940s, reports of its application for soft tissue augmentation began to surface.[4] Over the subsequent decades, the widespread use of various silicone oils for augmentation continued, unfortunately without common standards regarding sterility, purity, injection protocol, injection site, or injection volume.

One of the major historical difficulties in analyzing "silicone" as an augmenting agent is that an unknown and likely large proportion of substances claiming to be silicone have been adulterated, impure, or other substances entirely. Although highly purified, 350- and 1,000-cs products intended for injection into the human body were not introduced until the late 1960s and 1990s, respectively, and various substances masquerading as "silicone" have been injected for

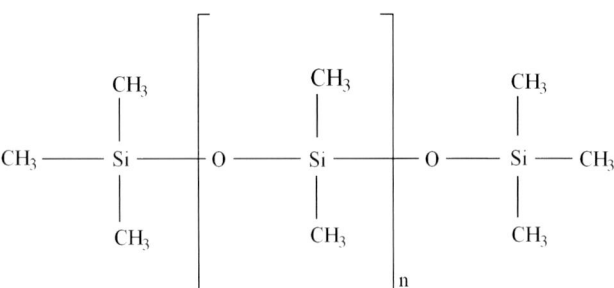

FIG. 8.1. *Linear molecular structure of polydimethylsiloxane. Repeating dimethylsiloxane units are flanked by terminal trimethylsiloxane units.*

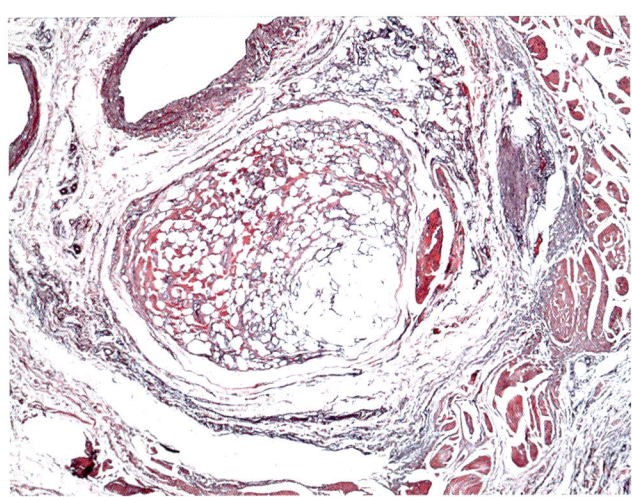

FIG. 8.2.   *Histology of silicone at eighteen years, showing round to oval spaces surrounded by dense fibrosis (courtesy of Drs. Sol W. Balkin and W. Dean Wallace).*

the past fifty to sixty years, at times with disastrous consequences. Indeed, liquid silicone was purposefully adulterated with vegetable oils for a brief period in an attempt to limit product migration, but this practice was stopped after frequent complications. Even products labeled as "medical-grade" silicone have not historically been regulated or ensured. A 1989 analysis of six "medical-grade" silicone oils commonly used for injection revealed six different products of variable viscosity, each with significant amounts of elemental impurities and low–molecular weight adulterants.[5]

Before the arrival of bovine collagen in the early 1980s, liquid silicone was the injectable filler of choice due to the natural texture and long-lasting results obtained with its use. However, with a growing number of critics and with mounting reports of complications such as granuloma formation and migration, its use declined alongside the widespread adoption of collagen as an alternative filler. Although in the early 1990s the Food and Drug Administration (FDA) banned the use of LIS for cosmetic implantation, legal use for this purpose was restored in 1997 with the passage of the US FDA Modernization Act,

which reaffirmed the physician's right to employ approved medical devices in an off-label manner. That same year, the FDA approved Silikon-1000 (Alcon, Fort Worth, TX) for intraocular retinal detachment, and hence, the use of approved products off-label legally resumed. The FDA has since clarified that off-label injection of approved products is legal as long as it is based on the unique needs of the patient and is not advertised or marketed for that purpose.[3,6] Furthermore, in 2001 and 2003, the FDA agreed to allow limited clinical studies investigating the use of approved silicone oils for the cosmetic improvement of nasolabial folds, labiomental folds, mid-malar depressions, and HIV-associated facial lipoatrophy. These studies are currently underway.

Advocates and critics of LIS have debated the merits and faults of LIS for over two decades, with each side basing their position largely on anecdotal data.[7] Critics maintain that LIS is an inherently unpredictable implant, laden with potential complications. Advocates, on the other hand, maintain that the product is extremely safe and beneficial when three tenets of treatment are strictly adhered to. First, only FDA-approved products intended for injection into the human body should be used. Second, the microdroplet serial puncture technique must be exclusively employed. Third, a protocol involving limited per-session injection volumes, spaced over multiple injection sessions, with adequate intersession spacing, must be followed.

Because the history of LIS has been confounded by reports of complications emanating from injection of unknown or impure substances, we assert that a more accurate profile of LIS as an augmenting agent may be attained by considering the growing data and experience obtained with highly purified LIS intended for injection into the human body. For the past five years, clinical trials have been underway with the newer generation of liquid silicones. These studies have so far demonstrated an excellent profile of safety and efficacy. The ongoing collection of objective data and longer term follow-up are necessary to provide clarity into the true risks and benefits of soft tissue augmentation with the modern silicones.

PATIENT SELECTION

Although LIS currently has no FDA-approved cosmetic indications, it may be effectively employed off-label for the augmentation of nasolabial folds, labiomental folds (so-called "marionette lines"), mid-malar depressions, postsurgical defects, hemi-facial atrophy, lip atrophy, acne scarring, age-related atrophy of the hands, corns and calluses of the feet, healed neuropathic foot ulcers, and HIV-associated or age-related facial lipoatrophy.[6] However, it is specifically contraindicated for injection into breasts, eyelids, bound-down scars, and actively inflamed sites. Nor should it be injected into patients with dental caries, chronic bacterial sinusitis, or those who may be subject to occupational or recreational facial trauma, such as in contact sports. The safety of LIS has not been studied in pregnant women and as such is contraindicated in this condition.

Furthermore, serious consideration must be given to the longevity of results obtained with LIS. Although, at the outset, those fillers with longer durations of action might seem clearly preferred to temporary fillers, this is not always the case. When evaluating the patient and treatment area, the possibility that aesthetic goals might change over time must be considered in light of the permanent nature of augmentation. Additionally, an undesired outcome will not likely diminish with time and may be difficult to correct. As previously mentioned, the best candidates for LIS have clear insight into their treatment goals and the permanent nature of the product, in contrast to those who seek immediate correction or temporary augmentation.

BENEFITS

With an increasing number of products for tissue augmentation available, the physician may now choose from a range of injectables with distinctive treatment profiles and varying durations. In the opinion of numerous skilled practitioners, many of whom have published their long-term experience, LIS is an exceptional agent for the treatment of certain types of acne scars (Figure 8.3A,B), rhytids, and HIV-associated facial lipoatrophy (Figures 8.4A,B and 8.5A,B).[8–11] Barnett has reported his thirty-year experience treating thousands of patients for various types of acne scarring with superb, persistent results, no significant adverse reactions, and very few incidents of overcorrection necessitating minor correction such as shave excision or corticosteroid injection.[9] When treating broad-based, depressed acne scars, LIS is the only augmenting agent that has been shown to achieve both corrective precision and permanence.

One of the foremost uses of all fillers to date has been augmentation of the age-related changes of the lower face, including nasolabial folds, labiomental folds, and mid-malar depressions. When appropriately employed, LIS has demonstrated merit in these areas as well, with an expected 30–90 percent improvement dependent on the depth of original depression. When the desired augmentative result is obtained, permanence is certainly a positive attribute in this area. However, notwithstanding the substantial and encouraging long-term experience of many accomplished injectors, we currently advocate that long-term safety data be further demonstrated through rigorous clinical trials before the widespread, routine use of LIS for acne scarring and rhytids.

On the other hand, investigational studies of the correction of HIV-associated facial lipoatrophy with 1,000 cs LIS are well underway, currently with outstanding five-year results. The poor body image,

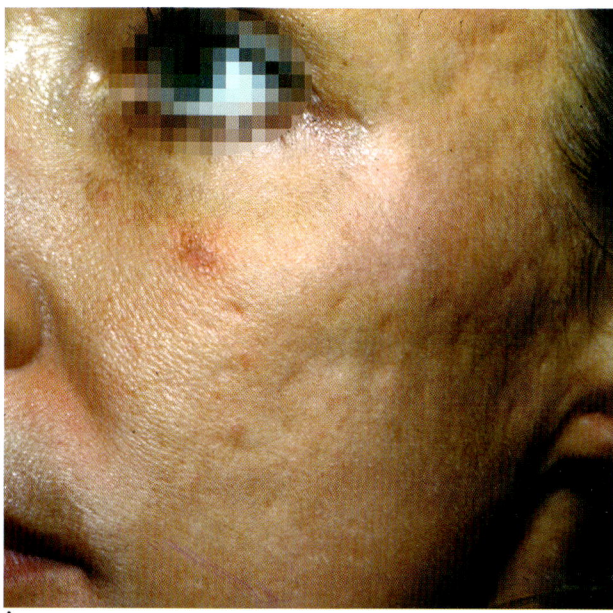
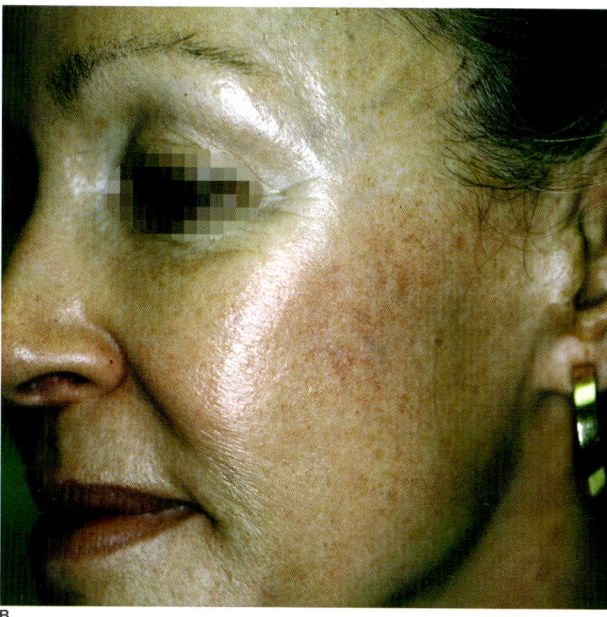

FIG. 8.3. *Long-term correction of facial acne scarring with LIS. (A) Pretreatment and (B) thirty-year follow-up (courtesy of Drs. Jay G. Barnett and Channing R. Barnett).*

lowered self-esteem, depression, and social and career barriers known to occur with HIV-associated facial lipoatrophy make it a significant therapeutic target. Furthermore, the permanence, natural texture in vivo, and high cost-to-benefit ratio of LIS make it an ideal augmentative agent for the correction of this potentially stigmatizing condition. To

date, over 700 patients with HIV lipoatrophy have been treated with Silikon-1000 by one of the authors (D. J.), with excellent results and without adverse events beyond the expected transient effects typically associated with any injection. A cohort of seventy-seven of these subjects was also analyzed to determine the number of treatments, amount of LIS,

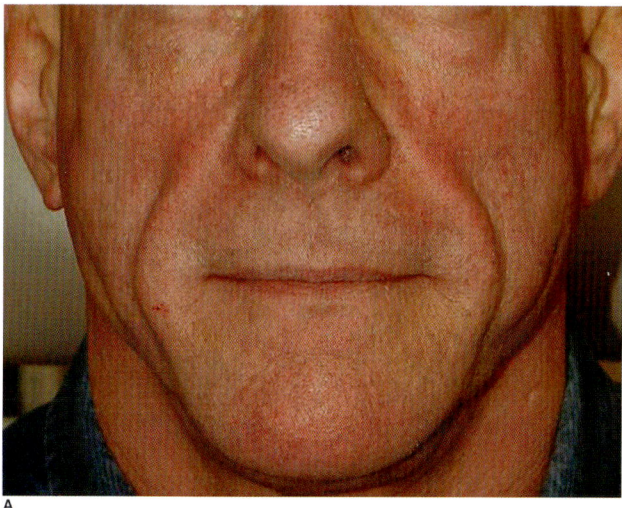
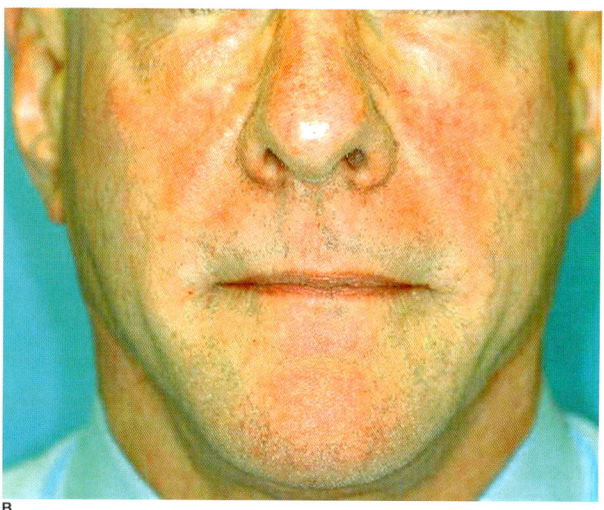

FIG. 8.4. *Correction of Stage 2 HIV-associated facial lipoatrophy, before (A) and after (B) six treatments with 10.5 mL total (courtesy of Blackwell Publishing[12]).*

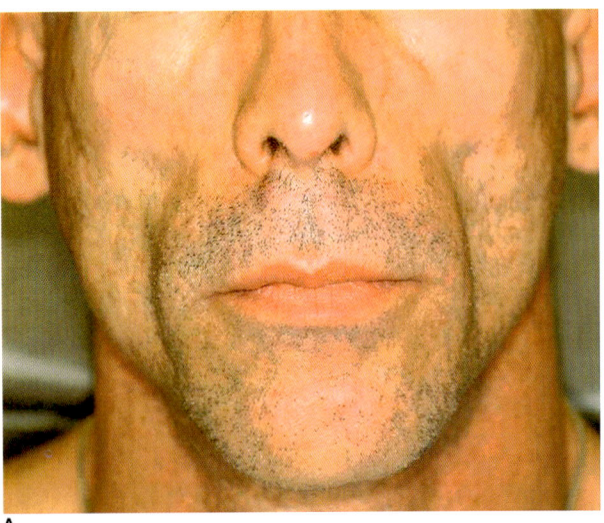
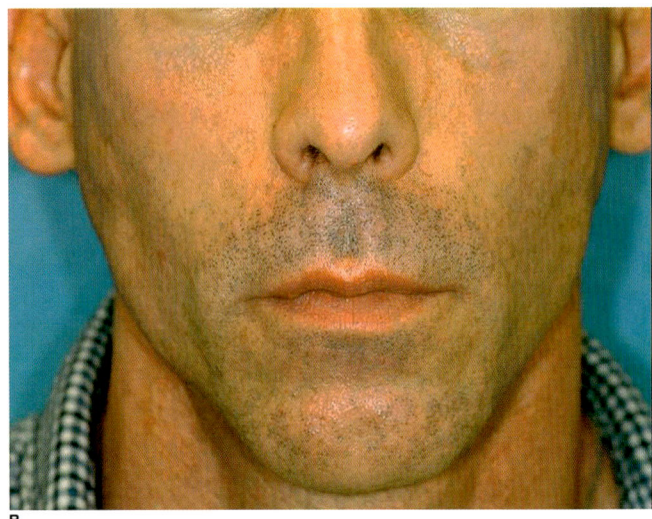

A   B

FIG. 8.5. Correction of Stage 3 HIV-associated facial lipoatrophy, before (A) and after (B) six treatments with 17 mL total (courtesy of Blackwell Publishing[12]).

and time required to reach the desired correction.[12] Each factor directly related to the initial degree of lipoatrophy severity ($p < 0.0001$) as determined by Carruthers' Facial Lipoatrophy Severity Scale.[13,14]

INSTRUMENTATION

The first precept of proper treatment with LIS is that only approved, highly purified silicone intended for injection into the human body be used. Although the 350 cs (approved in Europe) and the much more viscous 5,000 cs Adatosil (Bausch & Lomb, Rochester, NY) (approved in the United States) oils have been used with good results, the authors prefer Silikon-1000, currently the only FDA-approved 1,000 cs silicone oil (Figure 8.6). Because small volumes of LIS are to be injected in a given session, and precise microdroplet amounts must be dispensed, low-volume syringes are preferred. A 0.3-cc insulin syringe may be used, but it must be backloaded with product. The authors prefer a 1.0-cc Becton Dickinson Luer-Lok™ syringe, into which 0.5 cc of LIS may be drawn with sterile technique through a sixteen-gauge needle. Accurate flow of product and minimal patient discomfort are then achieved by injecting through a metal-hub twenty-seven-gauge needle. Additionally, the comfort of the injector may be improved by placing a 0.5-inch–inner diameter rubber electrical bushing over the barrel of the 1.0-cc

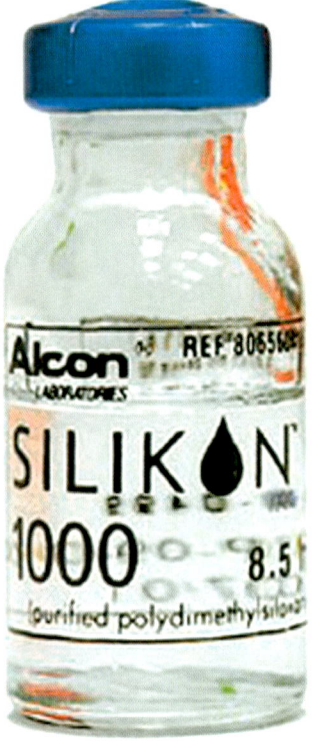

FIG. 8.6. Silikon-1000, currently the only FDA-approved 1,000 cs silicone oil (courtesy of Dr. David Duffy).

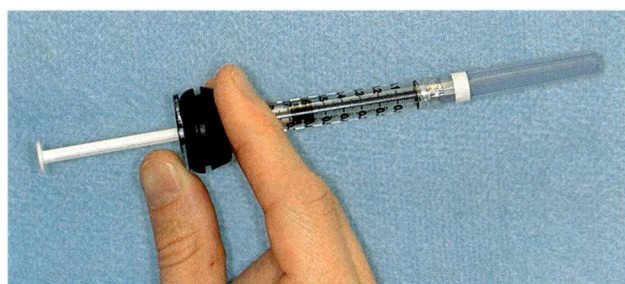

FIG. 8.7. *Rubber bushing used over the syringe for injector comfort (courtesy of Blackwell Publishing[19]).*

syringe to provide padding for the injector's second and third fingers (Figure 8.7). These may be purchased from a local hardware store and autoclaved for sterility.

PATIENT PREPARATION

In addition to understanding the risks and alternatives of treatment, patients must also accept the off-label and permanent nature of LIS. A detailed, written informed consent is of paramount importance before treatment. Additionally, high-quality pretreatment photographs should be taken. Patients should avoid any medications, vitamins, or supplements that may increase the risk of bleeding or bruising with treatment such as aspirin, nonsteroidal anti-inflammatory medications, anticoagulants, or vitamin E.

All makeup should be thoroughly removed before injection. The skin is then washed with an antibacterial cleanser and prepped with a povidone–iodine antiseptic. With the patient seated under adequate lighting, the areas to be treated are outlined with a fine-tipped surgical marking pen (Figure 8.8). Marking a seated patient in both the smiling and the resting facial positions is crucial to obtaining a desirable aesthetic result, particularly when treating the mid-malar areas in HIV-associated facial lipoatrophy. Overcorrection of these areas may result in a "chipmunk" type of appearance upon smiling and is to be avoided. After marking is complete, topical lidocaine is applied to the treatment areas. Thirty

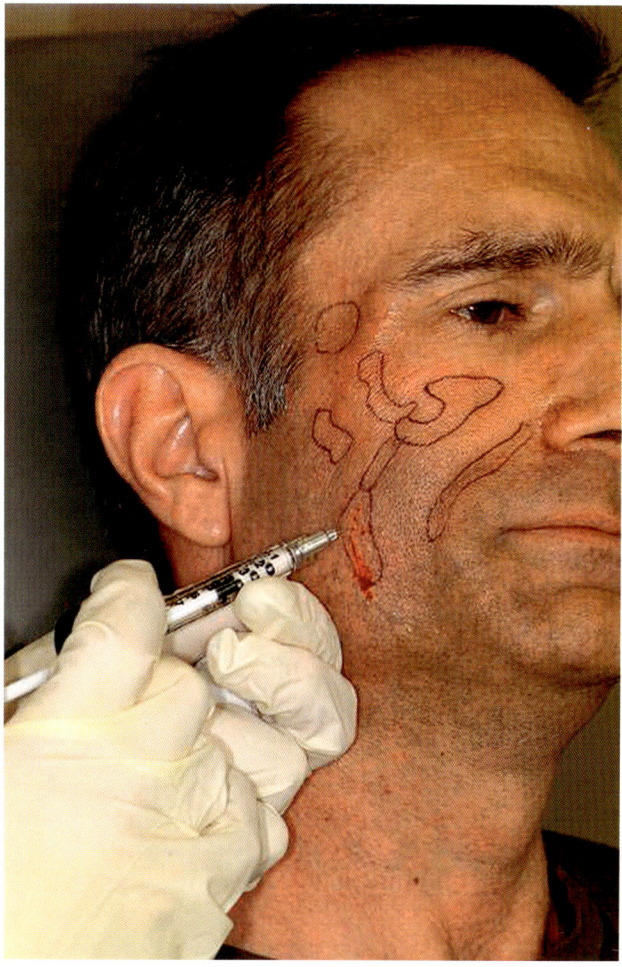

FIG. 8.8. *Patient marked for injection while in the seated position (courtesy of Blackwell Publishing[19]).*

to sixty minutes later, the anesthetic is gently wiped away with clean gauze so as to leave the physician's markings, and the treatment is begun.

INJECTION TECHNIQUE

The second precept of appropriate LIS protocol is that it should only be injected with the microdroplet serial puncture technique, as described by Orentreich.[3] Any other injection technique significantly increases the risk of complications such as beading, overcorrection, and product migration. A microdroplet is defined as 0.005–0.01 mL of product. The significance of the microdroplet is that it creates a very large surface area as compared to volume, which is important for two reasons: Foremost, a larger surface area to volume ratio effectively allows the microdroplet to be anchored into place by the ensuing fibroplasia that occurs around it. With larger macrodroplets, defined as >0.01 mL, encapsulation may not be sufficient to prevent product migration. Additionally, a larger surface area to volume ratio allows for a greater amount of fibroplasia, and thus augmentation, per unit volume. This notion is based on the principle that a given volume of LIS dispersed into many microdroplets provides for a greater surface area than would be provided by fewer, larger droplets. Because fibroplasia, or augmentation by the deposition of newly formed collagen, occurs on the surface of the LIS microdroplet, maximizing the surface area of injected product effectively maximizes the degree of augmentation.

The target of LIS deposition is the immediate subdermal plane or deeper. The location of this plane will vary according to treatment area but may generally be found approximately 5 mm below the skin surface. A slight decrease in resistance may often be felt as the needle enters the subdermal plane. The needle should be inserted at 2- to 5-mm intervals along the skin surface at the optimal angle for penetration and deposition into the subdermal plane. The optimal angle will vary with the anticipated depth of LIS placement. For areas where deeper placement is desired, a more oblique (approaching perpendicular to the skin surface) angle of insertion is best, whereas a more acute (approaching parallel to the skin surface) angle of insertion works best for more superficial deposition. One must exercise caution not to manipulate the plunger during insertion and withdrawal of the needle through the dermis, so as to avoid LIS deposition at the dermal level. Intradermal injection should be carefully avoided, particularly over bony structure, as an unfavorable "beading" effect may occur. Rarely, practiced injectors may use dermal deposition of LIS to achieve an augmentative effect in certain acne scars

and rhytids that lack dermal thickness, but this technique should be used only by the highly experienced.

Intentional overcorrection with LIS is also to be avoided. Because fibroplasia serves as a major mechanism of augmentation, and this process occurs over several weeks after implantation, the best results will be reached by undercorrection with serial injections spaced adequately over time. The per-session volume and total volume of LIS to be used are dependent on the total treatment area, pretreatment degree of lipoatrophy, if applicable, and desired level of augmentation. We recommend that per-session volumes range from approximately 0.5 cc of LIS for smaller treatment areas such as nasolabial folds to no more than 2.0 cc for larger areas such as facial lipoatrophy. Such per-session volumes allow around 100–200 individual injections with microdroplet deposition at 2- to 5-mm intervals, allowing a large treatment area to be covered in a single session if necessary. Importantly, greater correction should be achieved over time rather than with larger per-session volumes. In general, multiple passes over the same treatment area in a single session should also be avoided, although experienced injectors may sometimes make a second pass at a different subcutaneous level.

At least one-month interval between treatment sessions of the same area should occur to allow adequate time for collagen deposition and maximum augmentative effect. If a different area is being treated, however, it may be treated sooner. Although intervals longer than one month are acceptable as well, the time required to achieve the final end point will be prolonged. As the treatment end point approaches, the volume of LIS injected per session should diminish, and longer intervals between treatments should be planned. Intervals on the order of every two to six months are appropriate in the late treatment period to allow for delayed fibroplasia, during which continued treatment might result in overcorrection.

SIDE EFFECTS AND COMPLICATIONS

The side effects commonly associated with all injectable fillers may be expected with LIS as well. Generally, mild pain upon needle insertion is satisfactorily controlled with pretreatment topical anesthetics. If necessary, pretreatment with oral analgesics and nerve blocks may help supplement pain control in certain treatment areas or in those patients with a low pain tolerance. Mild postinjection edema is common and resolves within several hours to a few days. Postinjection edema may even produce a transient correction predictive of final optimal correction. Temporary ecchymosis is also a common side effect due to the large number of puncture sites necessary with the microdroplet technique. Additionally, the vascularity of the underlying tissue and the surface anticoagulant property of LIS may contribute to transitory bruising. Prolonged manual pressure may be employed in those patients who have not interrupted their anticoagulant treatment before injection to reduce the incidence and extent of ecchymosis. Makeup may also be applied to conceal postinjection ecchymosis. Tissue ischemia due to vascular injury or intravascular deposition has not been reported in the modern era using the highly purified 1,000 cs silicone oils with the microdroplet technique. However, such complications have been reported with other fillers and are a theoretical risk with silicone as well.

Discoloration is also a potential side effect of LIS. Moderate erythema may occasionally occur after injection. As a rule, it resolves after a few hours. Rarely, persistent erythema is observed, and it may be treated with a pulsed dye laser or topical and intralesional corticosteroids. Postinflammatory hyperpigmentation rarely occurs with LIS, manifesting as brown, yellow, or blue discoloration. Such discoloration has also been noted to occur more often with too superficial, dermal placement of LIS.

Detailed pretreatment photographs are important for discerning any dyschromia present before injection with LIS.

Dermal injection may be associated with other complications as well. If silicone is placed too superficially, the resulting fibroplastic collagen deposition may clinically result in "beading," defined as small 1- to 5-mm firm papules that may be visualized without palpation. Beading may rarely occur even when LIS is placed at the appropriate level in the subcutis. In some cases, beading will be temporary and will resolve without treatment over several months, but this is the exception. More often, beading will necessitate treatment with intralesional corticosteroids, low-power electrodessication, punch excision, dermabrasion, or tangential shave excision.

GRANULOMATOUS AND INFLAMMATORY REACTIONS

Much has been written in the literature about the granulomatous inflammatory reaction to injected "silicone," sometimes labeled with the misnomer "siliconoma." Yet careful scrutiny of these reports reveals that the presence of pure, unadulterated LIS, like that seen with the modern products approved by the FDA for injection into the human body, has not been conclusively established in the majority of reports. Additionally, such granulomas have rarely been reported when using appropriate products in the appropriate location with the microdroplet serial puncture technique. Rather, such cases fall into four causal categories: overinjection, injection into contraindicated sites, injection of impure material, or injection of substances of unknown chemical composition. Discretion must be exercised when evaluating reports of granulomatous reactions to "silicone," as many substances inappropriately masquerade under this title. Reflexion electron microscopy (REM) and electron dispersing X-ray

(EDX) technologies have been described as tools that may help determine the presence of silicone oil in reported complications, but these tools are not able to establish the purity of LIS or rule out the possibility of coexisting adulterants.[15] The authors assert that a prudent approach involves evaluating the recent generation of highly purified products in carefully controlled investigational studies on their own merits, separately from anecdotal complications involving both the less rigorously regulated formulations that preceded them and the uncontrolled substances that continue to be injected in an illicit manner.

Very rarely, experienced injectors using purified LIS have reported the occurrence of focal, indurated, chronic inflammatory nodules and plaques several months to years after treatment.[7] Similar reactions have been described with other long-term and permanent fillers such as polymethylmethacrylate and polylactic acid.[16,17] These well-demarcated areas of edema, with or without erythema, are estimated to occur with LIS once every 5,000–10,000 treatment sessions,[3] although they have not yet been reported with the newer generation of silicones available since the 1990s. Microscopic investigation of these complications has revealed a nonspecific, chronic inflammatory infiltrate, and intradermal testing with LIS, when performed, has been negative.[3] The reactions are noted to be localized within a given patient, leaving the majority of the treatment area uninvolved.

Such reactions are thought to be immune mediated, but the mechanism and causative factors remain uncertain. Because many of these reactions are frequently preceded by an infection at a nearby or distant site, one leading concept is that implanted LIS serves as a nidus for bacterial infection.[7] It is theorized that microorganisms from separate infectious processes, such as sinusitis, otitis, furunculosis, or a dental abscess, may encounter the silicone microdroplet either through direct extension or via the circulation. The LIS then acts as a colonized foreign body, capable of inducing a host inflammatory reaction in the immunocompetent patient. Furthermore, some postulate that immunocompromised patients who receive LIS may be at risk for this type of chronic focal inflammatory complication for an extended period after treatment if host immune function returns. The prototype for this would be the HIV patient who received LIS for facial lipoatrophy and later experienced immune restoration due to antiretroviral medications. Although such a concern has conceptual merit, this phenomenon has not been observed in the practice of one of us (D. J.) with extensive experience treating immunocompromised patients with LIS.

Duffy has superbly put forth the possible consequences of such a hypothetical immunopathogenic mechanism, including the prospective delayed host response.[7] He has also highlighted the potential effects of bacterial biofilms on LIS microdroplets.

Although granulomatous and inflammatory complications have so far proven to be negative on bacterial culture, this could be explained by the conversion of bacteria from a planktonic state to a biofilm state. A biofilm colony is one in which individual organisms are encased in a polysaccharide matrix and are not amenable to culture. Such a biofilm state might also portend resistance to clearance by antibiotics and frequent recurrence of inflammatory lesions. To be certain, all permanent implants, including LIS, should be considered contraindicated in those with evident or occult infections. In the literature, granulomatous and inflammatory reactions have been reported to respond within weeks to various treatments, including intralesional corticosteroids, oral tetracycline-class antibiotics, and etanercept.[18]

Migration, or "drift" of silicone along tissue planes to distant body sites, has been a documented complication when large boluses are injected since the early days of its use.[7] In contrast, it has been recognized since the 1960s that small aliquots injected over several sessions avoid this complication. In spite of this knowledge, migration of inappropriately large injection volumes of LIS is still occasionally reported, usually appearing when injections are illicitly given by a nonphysician outside of the medical setting.

SUMMARY

As the armamentarium of soft tissue–augmenting agents expands, LIS retains a unique and effective treatment profile when appropriately employed by an experienced injector using the microdroplet serial puncture technique. Although it is effective for the correction of various facial atrophies and deformities, currently its greatest application is for the permanent correction of HIV-associated facial lipoatrophy.

Although LIS has generated ample controversy in the past, the modern, highly purified silicone oils continue to be studied in controlled clinical settings and have so far proven to be extremely safe agents that warrant distinction from their predecessors. Yet it should be noted that complications may still occur and may be more difficult to treat due to the permanent nature of the product. For this reason, LIS should only be considered in appropriate patients who have had full disclosure as to the off-label nature of its use and adequate informed consent. When all criteria are met, LIS may be one of the most cost-effective and natural fillers available, and continued studies are ongoing to further examine both long-term safety and efficacy.

REFERENCES

1. Diamond B., Hulka B., Kerkvliet N., Tugwell P. Summary of report of national science panel: silicone breast implants in relation to connective tissue diseases and immunologic dysfunction (1998). http://www.fjc.gov/BREIMLIT/SCIENCE/summary.htm, accessed May 15, 2007.

2. Wallace W.D., Balkin S.W., Kaplan L., Nelson S.D. The histological host response of liquid silicone injections for prevention of pressure-related ulcers of the foot: a 38-year study. *Journal of the American Podiatric Medical Association* **94** (2004), pp. 550–557.

3. Orentreich D.S. Liquid injectable silicone: techniques for soft tissue augmentation. *Clinics in Plastic Surgery* **27** (2000), pp. 595–612.

4. Klein A.W. Skin filling: collagen and other injectables of the skin. *Dermatologic Clinics* **19** (2001), pp. 491–508.

5. Parel J.M. Silicone oils: physiochemical properties. In *Retina*, vol. 3, ed. Glaser B.M., Michels R.G. (St. Louis, MO: Mosby, 1989), pp. 261–277.

6. Orentreich D.S., Jones D.H. Liquid injectable silicone. In *Soft Tissue Augmentation*, ed. Carruthers J., Carruthers A. (New York, NY: Elsevier, 2005), pp. 77–91.

7. Duffy D.M. Liquid silicone for soft tissue augmentation: histological, clinical, and molecular perspectives. In *Tissue Augmentation in Clinical Practice*, 2nd edn., ed. Klein A. (New York, NY: Taylor & Francis, 2006), pp. 141–237.

8. Balkin S.W. Injectable silicone and the foot: a 41-year clinical and histologic history. *Dermatologic Surgery* **31** (11 pt. 2) (2005), pp. 1555–1559.

9. Barnett J.G., Barnett C.R. Treatment of acne scars with liquid silicone injections: 30-year perspective. *Dermatologic Surgery* **31** (11 pt. 2) (2005), pp. 1542–1549.

10. Duffy D.M. Liquid silicone for soft tissue augmentation. *Dermatologic Surgery* **31** (11 pt. 2) (2005), pp. 1530–1541.

11. Jones D. HIV facial lipoatrophy: causes and treatment options. *Dermatologic Surgery* **31** (11 pt. 2) (2005), pp. 1519–1529.

12. Jones D.H., Carruthers A., Orentreich D., Brody H.J., Lai M.Y., Azen S., Van Dyke G.S. Highly purified 1000 centistoke oil for treatment of HIV-associated facial lipoatrophy. *Dermatologic Surgery* **30** (2004), pp. 1276–1286.

13. Jones D. Treatment of HIV facial lipoatrophy. Presentation at the ASDS (American Society of Dermatologic Surgery)-ACMMSCO (American College of Mohs Micrographic Surgery and Cutaneous Oncology) Combined Annual Meeting (Oct. 31 – Nov. 3, 2002), Chicago, IL.

14. James J., Carruthers A., Carruthers J. HIV-associated facial lipoatrophy. *Dermatologic Surgery* **28** (2002), pp. 979–986.

15. Lloret P., Espana A., Leache A., Bauza A., Fernandez-Galar M., Idoate M.A., Plewig G., Weber L. Successful treatment of granulomatous reactions secondary to injection of esthetic implants. *Dermatologic Surgery* **31**(4) (2005), pp. 486–490.

16. Gelfer A., Carruthers A., Carruthers J., Jang F., Bernstein S.C. The natural history of polymethylmethacrylate microspheres granulomas. *Dermatologic Surgery* **33**(5) (2007), pp. 614–620.

17. Wildemore J.K., Jones D.H. Persistent granulomatous inflammatory response induced by injectable poly-L-lactic acid for HIV lipoatrophy. *Dermatologic Surgery* **32**(11) (2006), pp. 1407–1409.

18. Pasternack F.R., Fox L.P., Engler D.E. Silicone granulomas treated with etanercept. *Archives of Dermatology* **141**(1) (2005), pp. 13–15.

19. Prather C.L., Jones D.H. Liquid injectable silicone for soft tissue augmentation. *Dermatologic Therapy.*

Chapter 9

ADVANTA EXPANDED POLYTETRAFLUOROETHYLENE IMPLANTS

by

Kelley Pagliai Redbord, MD and
C. William Hanke, MD, MPH, FACP

INTRODUCTION

The skin's natural aging process manifests itself in the form of contour changes, wrinkles, the depletion of subcutaneous fat, and the loss of dermal collagen and elastin. Today's patients are seeking skin rejuvenation to achieve a natural and youthful appearance through minimally invasive procedures with no downtime. Thinning of the lips and deepening of the nasolabial folds and marionette lines are common manifestations of the aging process. Despite multiple treatment modalities and advances in cosmetic surgery, long-lasting, natural-looking augmentation in these areas continues to present a challenge. Available since January 1, 2001, Advanta expanded polytetrafluoroethylene (ePTFE) implants (Ocean Breeze Surgical, Amherst, NH) have been used successfully for augmentation of thinning lips, deep nasolabial folds, and marionette lines without the risk, recovery time, and expense of major surgery.

DESCRIPTION OF THE ADVANTA ePTFE IMPLANT

Advanta ePTFE implants are an expanded porous polytetrafluoroethylene material with a unique dual-porosity structure.[1,2] ePTFE is a stable polymer of carbon atoms with a coating of fluorine atoms.[3] The unique dual-porosity structure has a soft high-porosity 100-μm central core surrounded by a smooth, medium-porosity 40-μm outer core. This unique dual-porosity concept promotes tissue integration, vascular ingrowth, and stability. This is critical in preventing migration and reducing shrinkage.[3] The dual-porosity structure is also responsible for a soft feel giving it natural-looking results.

Advanta ePTFE implants are available in sheets and geometrical shapes with and without reinforcement. The implants are either round or oval (Figure 9.1). Round implants are available in 2.5, 3.0, 4.0, 5.0, and 6.0 mm diameters with preattached stainless steel trocars and 4.0, 5.0, and 6.0 mm without

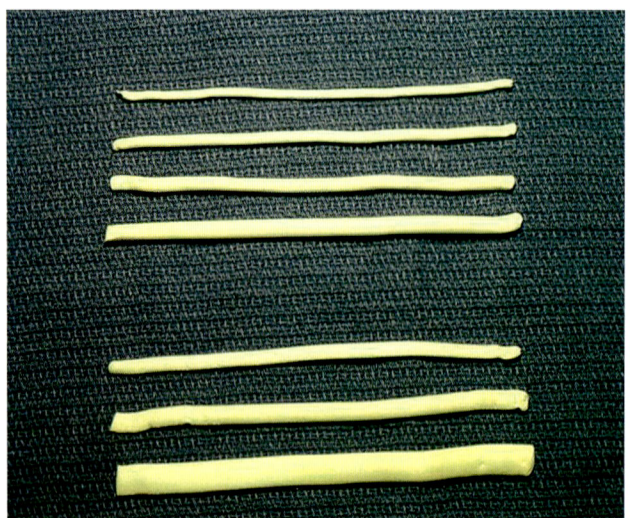

FIG. 9.1. *Advanta ePTFE implants are available in round (top three strips) or oval (bottom three strips) shapes in various diameters.*

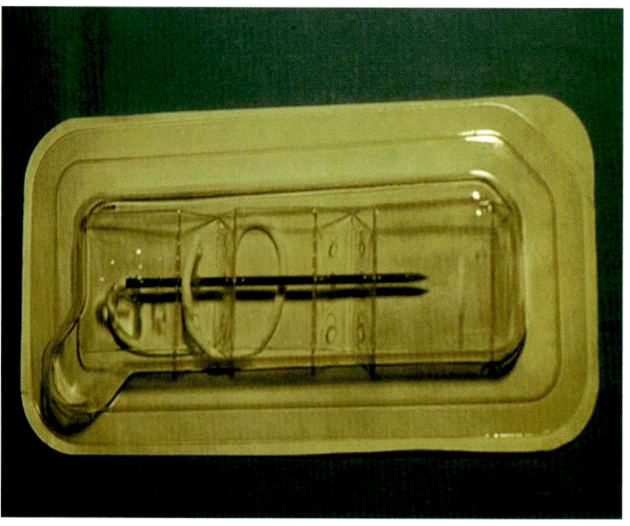

FIG. 9.2. *Advanta ePTFE round implants are available with or without preattached stainless steel trocars.*

preattached trocars (Figure 9.2). Oval implants are available in 3.2 × 5.4 mm, 3.5 × 6.5 mm, 4.5 × 6.5 mm, and 5.0 × 7.0 mm diameters with preattached stainless steel trocars and 3.0 × 4.2 mm, 3.2 × 5.4 mm, 3.5 × 6.5 mm, 4.5 × 6.5 mm, and 5.0 × 7.0 mm without preattached trocars. The implants are 15 cm in length to allow a single implant to be used for both nasolabial folds or both upper and lower lips in most patients.

INDICATIONS

Advanta ePTFE implants are indicated for augmentation of the facial area specifically the nasolabial folds, upper and lower lips, marionette lines, glabellar furrows, and other deep wrinkles and soft tissue defects.[1,4] It is not indicated for superficial fine lines.

CONTRAINDICATIONS

Advanta ePTFE implants are contraindicated for dermal placement and for temporomandibular joint reconstruction.[4] Implants should not be placed in infected areas. Relative contraindications include

patients with professional or vocational activities that require precise oral function.[5]

ePTFE implants should be used with caution in patients with autoimmune diseases or diabetes who may have abnormal wound healing. Similarly, ePTFE implants should be used with caution in patients with severe acne because of increased risk of infection.

IMPLANT PROCEDURE

Preoperative

Patients are instructed to wash the lower one-third of the face twice daily with chlorhexidine gluconate for two days preoperatively.[1] Oral antibiotics (i.e., cephalexin 500 mg twice a day) are taken one day preoperatively and continued for seven days. Thereafter, the dose is reduced to 250 mg twice daily for two more weeks. All anticoagulation agents including aspirin, nonsteroidal anti-inflammatory drugs, vitamin E, and other herbal agents are discontinued two weeks before the procedure. Patients are instructed to stop smoking ten days before and after the procedure.[2] Photographs should be obtained before beginning the treatment and at follow-up. Informed consent should be obtained

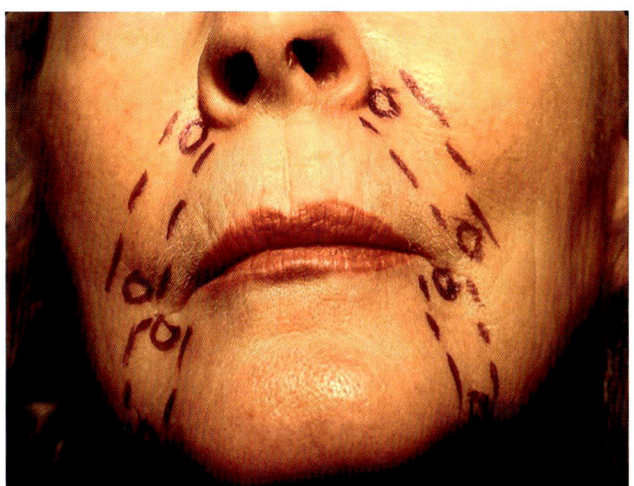

FIG. 9.3. *Before injection, facial landmarks are outlined for the placement of implants in the nasolabial folds and marionette lines. The circles indicate the sites for the stab incisions.*

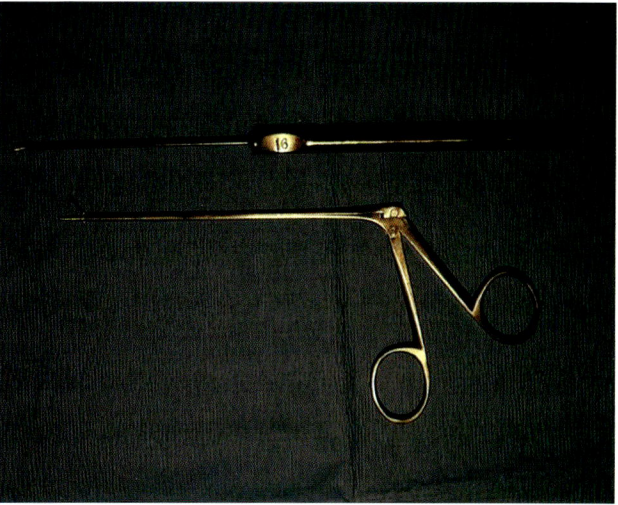

FIG. 9.4. *A 2.0-mm-diameter closed-neck dissector (top) with the V-shaped tip creates a subcutaneous tunnel for the implant. A Hartmann alligator forcep (bottom) with open jaws can be used to pull the implant through the tunnel.*

detailing the risks and benefits associated with the procedure. Skin testing is not required before use.

Select the appropriate size and shape of the Advanta ePTFE implant based on the soft tissue defect that is to be corrected. Oval implants are more commonly used to augment the nasolabial folds. Round, 3- to 4-mm-diameter, implants are most commonly used to augment the lips. Small-diameter oval or round implants can be used for the marionette lines and glabellar frown lines. For lip augmentation, the lip length should be measured with the mouth open to ensure correct length.[5] Failure to measure with the mouth open can result in too short an implant and suboptimal results.

Before injection, the skin is prepped with chlorhexidine gluconate and the soft tissue defect is outlined with a wax marking pencil with the patient in an upright position to accurately determine the natural skin folds (Figure 9.3). Sterile techniques are strictly followed and the implants are handled with sterile gloves.

Nasolabial Fold Augmentation

Anesthesia is obtained using infraorbital nerve blocks via the intraoral route using 1 percent lidocaine with 1:100,000 epinephrine.[1] The areas to be treated are also locally anesthetized with a small amount of lidocaine with epinephrine as needed for complete anesthesia. After injection of the local anesthesia, facial landmarks can be distorted. However, the areas to be treated have been previously outlined for precise planning purposes. Oval implants are most commonly used for the augmentation of nasolabial folds. A single 15-cm implant divided into half is of sufficient length to treat both nasolabial folds.

Small stab incisions are made at the superior and inferior nasolabial fold with a no. 11 scalpel blade that is widened by iris scissors. A 2.0-mm-diameter closed-neck dissector is inserted in the inferior incision and is pushed through to the superior incision in the subcutaneous plane (Figure 9.4). The dissector is removed through the inferior incision creating a subcutaneous tunnel for the implant.

For the round implant to be inserted, the attached cannula is advanced superiorly in the subcutaneous plane from the inferior incision and removed from above (Figure 9.5). The skin is molded to a natural contour over the implant. The implants should not demonstrate dimpling, which indicates superficial

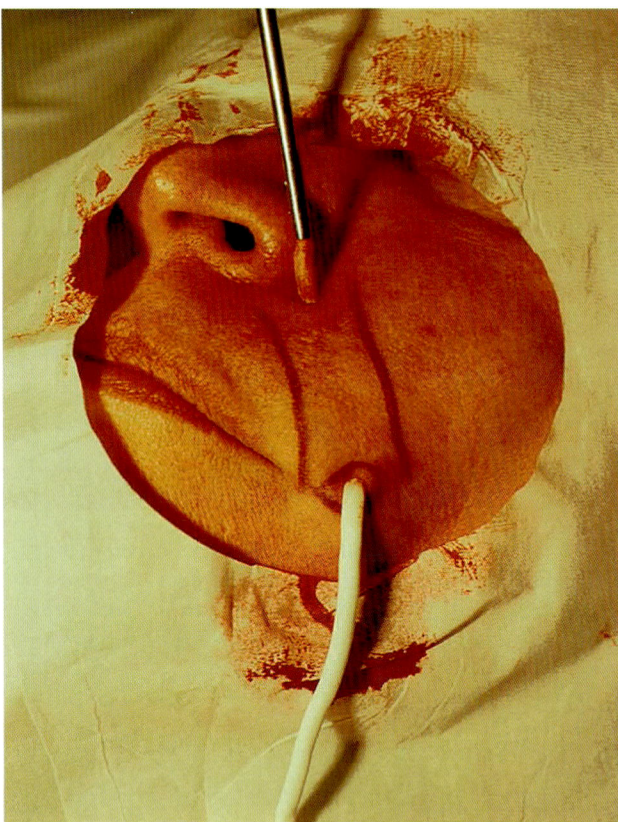

FIG. 9.5.   *Advanta ePTFE implant with a preattached stainless steel trocar is advanced superiorly in the subcutaneous plane from the inferior incision and removed from above.*

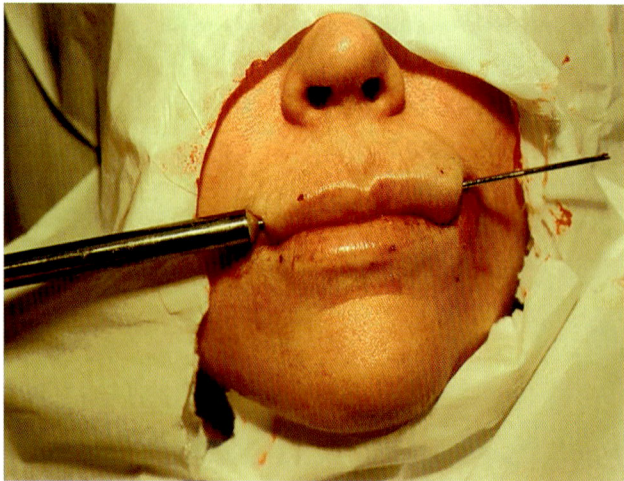

FIG. 9.6.   *The closed-neck dissector is advanced in a plane above the orbicularis muscle and removed.*

implantation. The implant ends are trimmed and the free ends buried using forceps. The small stab incisions are closed with 6–0 absorbable clear nylon suture. The oval implants do not always have an attached trocar. Therefore, after subcutaneous tunneling, a Hartmann alligator forcep (Anthony Products, Indianapolis, IN) is inserted in the inferior incision and pushed through in the subcutaneous plane to the superior incision (Figures 9.4 and 9.5). The implant is grasped with the alligator forceps and pulled through the tunnel.

Lip Vermilion Augmentation

Anesthesia is obtained using infraorbital and mental nerve blocks via the intraoral route using 1 percent lidocaine with 1:100,000 epinephrine.[1] The areas

to be treated are also locally anesthetized with approximately 10 cc of 0.5 percent lidocaine with 1:200,000 epinephrine as needed for complete anesthesia.

Upper lip augmentation is preferably performed before the lower. Three- or 4-mm round implants are most commonly used. Oval implants have a tendency to twist and are more difficult to orient.[2] A single 15-cm implant divided into half can be used to augment the entire upper and lower lips; however, the manufacturer suggests using separate implants for the upper and lower lips. Small vertical stab incisions are made 2–3 mm medial to each oral commissure into the vermilion with a no. 11 scalpel blade and widened with iris scissors. The closed-neck dissector is advanced in a plane above the orbicularis muscle and removed (Figure 9.6). If the plane is created too superficially, the implant will be visible, palpable, and unnatural.[5] If the plane is too deep, less augmentation will occur. The round implant with attached trocar is slowly advanced through the tunnel to avoid separation of the trocar from the implant. Care is taken to avoid the labial artery that is found in the posterior one-third of the lip. The skin is molded manually to a natural contour over the implant. Attempts to reconstruct the Cupid's bow are usually unnecessary and

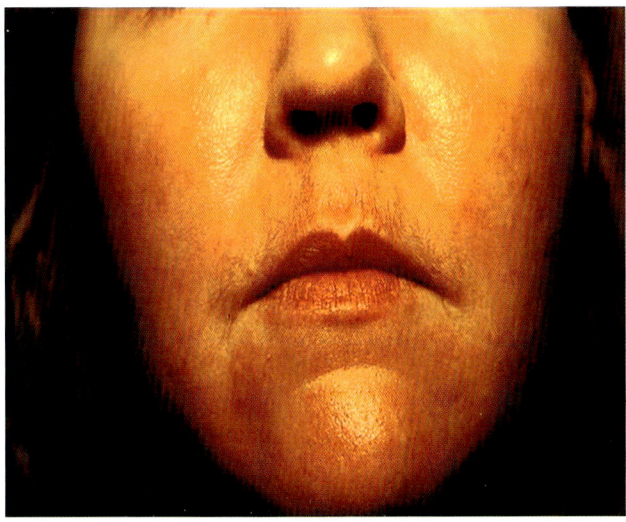

FIG. 9.7.   *A patient demonstrates thin lips and requests lip augmentation.*

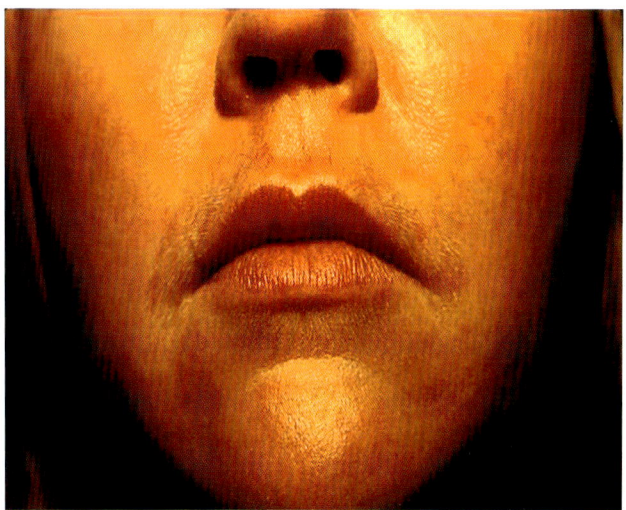

FIG. 9.8.   *Augmentation of both the upper and the lower lips after treatment with a 3.0-mm round Advanta ePTFE implant.*

may lead to suboptimal results. An injectable filler can be layered over the implant to define the Cupid's bow if desired.[2] The implant ends are trimmed and buried. The small stab incisions are closed with 6–0 absorbable clear nylon suture.

The implants are soft and are unnoticeable (even during kissing), which is a concern of patients receiving implants (Figures 9.7–9.10). There is no problem with normal oral function such as eating, speaking, or smiling.[6]

Postoperative

Application of ice packs to the nasolabial folds or lips is recommended for fifteen minutes every hour when

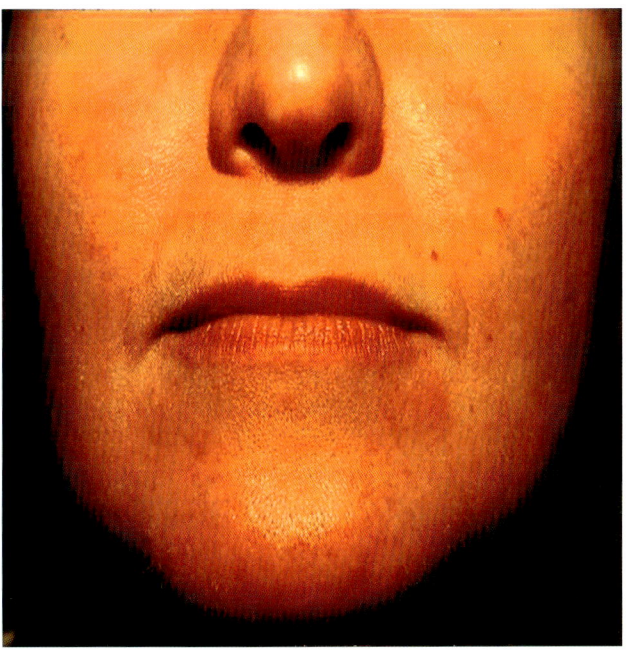

FIG. 9.9.   *A patient before augmentation demonstrating thin lips.*

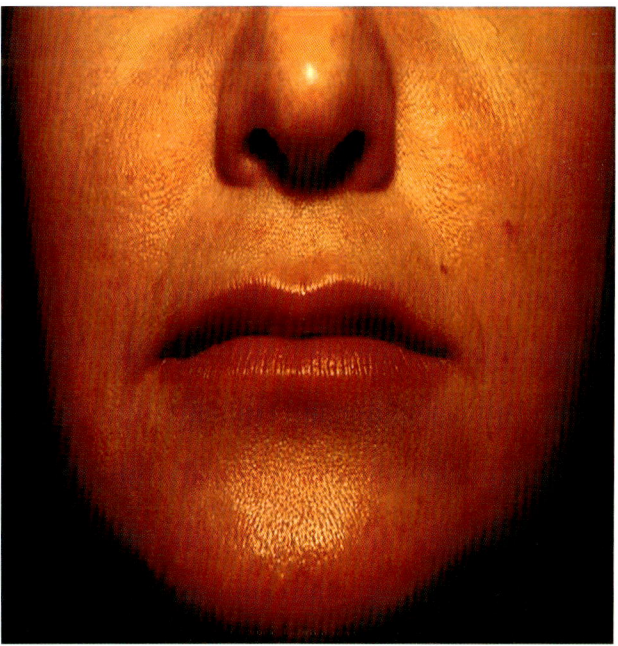

FIG. 9.10.   *Postaugmentation with a 3.0-mm round Advanta ePTFE implant into the upper and lower lips.*

the patient is awake over the next twelve to twenty-four hours to minimize bruising and swelling.[1] Swelling and bruising of the nasolabial folds are usually minimal, but the lips can swell considerably. Slight swelling is noticeable usually only to the patient for several weeks. Sutures are removed within three to four days. The patient is to refrain from heavy physical activity until suture removal, but normal activity such as brisk walking is allowed. Patients are instructed not to palpate the implants with their fingers or manipulate the implants with their tongue for several days.

COMPARISON TO OTHER TREATMENTS

There are many choices for patients seeking facial augmentation. Augmentation of the lips, nasolabial folds, and marionette lines can be achieved with degradable and nondegradable implant materials and injectable tissue fillers.[1] Patients with no history of augmentation may prefer a trial of a temporary filler to assess results and expectations. Degradable implant materials include collagen, hyaluronic acid, poly-L-lactic acid, calcium hydroxylapatite, and autologous fat.

Many patients are interested in a one-time permanent treatment and may prefer a nondegradable implant. Nonbiodegradable synthetic materials include silicone, Artecoll (Rofil Medical International, Breda, the Netherlands), Gore-Tex (WL Gore & Associates, Flagstaff, AZ), and Soft-Form (Collagen Corp., Palo Alto, CA). Silicone fluid is not approved by the US Food and Drug Administration (FDA) for cosmetic use. Artecoll, or multiple polymethylmethacrylate spheres suspended in bovine collagen, is approved for use in the United States, Europe, and Canada. It has a silicone-like effect and is injected at the junction of the dermis and subcutaneous fat.

ePTFE implants include Advanta, Gore-Tex, Soft-Form, and UltraSoft. In 1993, the US FDA approved Gore-Tex implants for facial augmentation. Gore-Tex, available since 1971, is an ePTFE

implant available in many shapes, sizes, and forms. Potential complications include extrusion, infection, migration, shrinkage, and scarring.[7] The lower porosity Gore-Tex implants show less tissue ingrowth than dual-porosity Advanta implants.[3] Gore-Tex SAM (Subcutaneous Augmentation Material) strands have the potential to become hard and uncomfortable with minimal tissue integration and stabilization. The manufacturer of Gore-Tex added silver and chlorhexidine to its ePTFE implants to minimize infection.[8] However, Gore-Tex departed from the ePTFE facial implant market at the end of 2006 and its products are no longer available. Soft-Form, introduced in 1997, is a hollow, tube-shaped ePTFE implant with a unique "no-touch" implantation technique for the treatment of deep facial furrows such as the nasolabial fold and lip augmentation. Potential complications include extrusion, infection, migration, shrinkage, and scarring.[9] It is a stiff implant without the feel of normal tissue. Given its small pore size, it has a higher risk of migration, hardening, and shrinkage than Advanta.[3,9] UltraSoft (Tissue Technologies Inc., San Francisco, CA), a thin-walled version of Soft-Form, is also available. Physician satisfaction with Gore-Tex, Soft-Form, and UltraSoft is low. One hundred percent of physicians surveyed by Cox in 2005 reported disappointment with the implants and noted revision rates of 5–100 percent.[10] Disappointment was due to the hardening of the implant, contraction with step-off deformities, and ability to see the implant through the skin. Physicians reported that Advanta ePTFE was superior to other available implants.

PATIENT SATISFACTION

Patient and physician satisfaction with the Advanta ePTFE implants is high.[1,2] Fezza reported experience with over fifty patients and found very high patient satisfaction.[2] Verret et al. treated 170 patients with 612 implants and found 14 patients or 8 percent dissatisfied with their implants but none were removed.[11] Patients previously treated with other ePTFE implants such as Gore-Tex or Soft-Form that were later replaced with Advanta implants reported higher satisfaction with the appearance and feel of their new implants.[3] Advanta ePTFE implants are soft and natural. The procedure is quick, the recovery rapid, and the results permanent.

COMPLICATIONS

Treatment-related complications from Advanta implants are uncommon with rates as low as 1.3 percent and include swelling, bruising, and infection.[1,8,11] No systemic complications from Advanta implants have been reported in the literature. Swelling and bruising are minimized if the precise technique is followed. Placement of the implants with a "single-pass" technique and advancing the trocar slowly minimizes trauma and limits postoperative bruising. Postoperative application of ice to the area is also helpful. Bruising is minimized by infiltration of local anesthesia to supplement the nerve block and by stopping all anticoagulant medications before the procedure. Infection can be prevented by using the proper sterile technique during implantation and prophylactic oral antibiotic use. Hanke reported three complications after implantation of sixty Advanta ePTFE in thirty patients.[1] One complication was bruising secondary to the patient taking aspirin, which resolved in five days; one complication was suspected infection requiring implant removal and subsequent replacement without complication; and the last complication was prolonged swelling that resolved with implant removal. Niamtu reported seventy-two Advanta implants in forty-four patients and found few complications.[5,6] He reported three infections; two of the three implants were replaced after the infection cleared. Several implants were too short for the treatment site. One mucous retention cyst developed from trauma to the minor salivary glands during implantation. Fezza reported two infections in fifty patients treated.[2] Truswell reported experience with 106 Advanta implants in forty-two patients and found three infections requiring removal and 1 implant requiring trimming for a better fit.[3] Rudolph et al. reported one case of delayed herpes simplex virus (HSV) infection after Gore-Tex threads were implanted.[12] HSV has not been reported with Advanta to date.

Other complications include inflammation, fistula formation, migration, extrusion, hematoma, induration, seroma formation, inadequate healing, and insufficient or exaggerated augmentation.[4] Migration and induration are rare, given the dual-porosity construct. Implantation erroneously into the dermis can lead to fistula formation, infection, extrusion, and induration.[4] If undercorrection is a concern, stacking implants is not a good corrective option as it gives an unnatural look. However, layering with an injectable filler over the implant can naturally augment the area for ideal correction.[2]

Although rare, complications can necessitate removal of the implants. Verret et al. reported experience with 612 implants and only 3 or 0.49 percent were removed.[11] The implants can be easily removed. However, given the extensive tissue integration from Advanta's dual-porosity structure, removal after 180 days may be more difficult necessitating longitudinal dissection along the implant.[1]

CONCLUSION

Advanta ePTFE implants are a safe, effective, and permanent option for facial volume augmentation of contour deficiencies due to aging. The implants provide a soft and natural-looking augmentation of the nasolabial folds, lips, marionette lines, glabella, and other soft tissue defects of the face. Training and experience in implantation is essential for the successful creation of a more youthful and natural appearance. Complications are rare, and removal of the implants is straightforward. Advanta ePTFE implants are another choice for patients seeking permanent facial augmentation.

REFERENCES

1. Hanke CW. A new ePTFE soft tissue implant for natural-looking augmentation of lips and wrinkles. *Dermatol Surg* 2002; **28**:901–8.

2. Fezza JP. Advanta implants. *Facial Plast Surg* 2004; **20**(2):185–9.

3. Truswell WH. Dual-porosity expanded polytetra-fluoroethylene soft tissue implant. *Arch Facial Plast Surg* 2002; **4**(2):92–7.

4. Atrium Medical Corporation, Hudson, NH. Advanta PTFE facial implants package insert. 2001.

5. Niamtu J III. Advanta ePTFE facial implants in cosmetic facial surgery. *J Oral Maxillofac Surg* 2006; **64**:543–9.

6. Niamtu J III. Who is still using lip implants? *Dermatol Surg* 2006; **32**(10):1302–4.

7. Sclafani AP, Thomas JR, Cox AJ, Cooper MH. Clinical and histologic response of subcutaneous expanded polytetrafluoroethylene (Gore-Tex) and porous high density polyethylene (Medpor) implants to acute and early infection. *Arch Otolaryngol Head Neck Surg* 1997; **123**:329–36.

8. Panossian A, Garner WL. Polytetrafluoroethylene facial implants: 15 years later. *Plast Reconstr Surg* 2004; **113**(1):347–9.

9. Brody HJ. Complications of expanded polytetrafluoro-ethylene (ePTFE) facial implant. *Dermatol Surg* 2001; **27**:792–4.

10. Cox SE. Who is still using expanded polytetrafluoro-ethylene? *Dermatol Surg* 2005; **31**:1613–5.

11. Verret DJ, Leach JL, Gilmore J. Dual-porosity expanded polytetrafluoroethylene implants for lip, nasolabial groove, and melolabial groove augmentation. *Arch Facial Plast Surg* 2006; **8**:423–5.

12. Rudolph CM, Mullegger RR, Schuller-Petrovic S, Kerl H, Soyer P. Unusual herpes simplex virus infection mimicking foreign body reaction after cosmetic lip augmentation with expanded polytetra-fluoroethylene threads. *Dermatol Surg* 2003; **29**:195–7.

Chapter 10

SCULPTRA

by

Cheryl Karcher, MD

INTRODUCTION

There has been a paradigm shift in cosmetic surgery. We are now replenishing volume that has been depleted in the facial region as opposed to removing excess skin that remains. Facial lipoatrophy is a facet of a more general condition, lipodystrophy. It is a symptom of various conditions that include congenital disorders, HIV-related therapies, and aging. Because facial lipoatrophy, regardless of cause, is a disfiguring condition that affects many people, several devices have been used in an attempt to provide aesthetic correction for this condition. Some of these injectable devices include fat, collagen, hyaluronic acids, calcium hydroxylapatite, silicones, poly-L-lactic acid (PLLA), and polymers such as polymethyl methacrylate and polyacrylamide. Sculptra is a synthetic, biodegradable, and biocompatible injectable composed of PLLA. This is one of the few substances approved in Europe and in the United States for correction of lipoatrophy that has pending cosmetic uses.[1,2]

Injectable PLLA is a new class of devices that provides a semipermanent option to correct the visible signs of facial lipoatrophy. Sculptra was approved with CE Mark certification under the trade name New-Fill in Europe. It has been estimated that 150,000 patients in over thirty countries have been treated with New-Fill since 1999. Sculptra has been used to increase the volume of depressed areas, such as skin creases, wrinkles, folds, and scars. In 2004, PLLA's approval was extended in Europe to include the large volume corrections of facial lipoatrophy. In the United States, injectable PLLA was approved by the FDA for the restoration and correction of facial lipoatrophy in patients with HIV in August 2004. In the United States, Sculptra Aesthetic was approved by the FDA in July 2009 for the correction of shallow to deep nasolabial folds (shallow lines), contour deficiencies, and other facial wrinkles that are treated with the appropriate injection technique in healthy patients. This device is unique as it results in neocollagenesis in the dermis and, therefore, requires a specific delivery technique for optimal results.[2]

SCULPTRA (PLLA) COMPOSITION

Sculptra is composed of microparticles of PLLA, a biocompatible, biodegradable, and synthetic polymer from the alpha-hydroxy-acid family. The final composition of Sculptra consists of 150 mg of PLLA, 90 mg of sodium carmellose, and 127.5 mg of apyrogenic mannitol in the freeze-dried form. The PLLA particles provide the durable attributes of Sculptra treatment. Raw material is milled, sieved, and sterilized before manufacture. PLLA microparticles are irregular in shape and have an average particle diameter of 40–63 μm. Polylactic acid is synthesized by esterification and polymerization of lactide monomers where the material is immunologically inert.[1,3] The amorphous crystalline structure and high molecular weight (>100,000 Da) of the product are responsible for the slow absorption when injected into the tissue. Once injected, 75 percent of the PLLA is broken down into CO_2 and H_2O. No allergy testing is required before use since PLLA is a synthetic material of nonanimal origin.[3]

PLLA has been widely used as a suture material for over forty years (Vicryl; Ethicon, Piscataway, NJ) as well as a vector for sustained release medications in other pharmaceutical products. Sodium carboxymethylcellulose is included as a suspending agent; it has an affinity for water to maintain even distribution of PLLA particles after reconstitution. It is "generally recognized to be safe" (GRAS) for use in food and is included in the FDA inactive ingredients guide for intradermal, intramuscular, intravenous, and subcutaneous injections. Sodium carboxymethylcellulose is also used as a thickening agent in foods, such as ice cream, and in several medical products such as eye drops and hydrocolloid dressing. Mannitol is included to enhance the lyophilization process. It produces a stiff, homogeneous cake and provides a suspension with an osmosity suitable for injection. An important property of sodium carboxymethylcellulose and mannitol is that they are both completely biodegradable.[1]

MECHANISM OF ACTION

The mechanism of action by which PLLA corrects facial volume deficiencies is not comprehensively understood. Several histological studies of PLLA injections in mice reported a pronounced tissue response. Investigators observed polylactides surrounded by vascularized connective tissue capsules, consisting of connective tissue cells with mononuclear macrophages, lymphocytes, foreign body cells, and mast cells after one month of implantation. Over time, the capsule surrounding the implants decreased in cell number, whereas thickness and collagen fibers increased. In general, PLLA was well tolerated by the tissue and no acute inflammation, abscess formation, or tissue necrosis was observed adjacent to the injection sites.[4]

Sculptra induces an immediate, local reaction that is followed by a progressive increase in volume. Within a few days, water absorption and the reduction of edema will result in a return to the baseline depression. Within several weeks of the injection, a natural, soft increase in dermal thickness due to neocollagenesis will begin to take shape. Larger volume defects may require additional treatment injections.[5]

It has been shown that PLLA has a rate of degradation that increases, associated with higher molecular weights. PLLA molecules with a higher molecular weight tend to degrade rapidly, falling to 3 percent of their initial weight six months after injection. One possibility of the rapid degradation may be due to the higher porosity with the higher molecular weight polymers. PLLA is degraded through enzymatic and nonenzymatic pathways.[6] In vitro degradation of PLLA involves hydrolysis of ester bonds that results in the formation of lactide monomers and oligomers and carboxylic acids, which catalyze the degradation process. As PLLA is degraded, trace amounts of polymerization initiators, such as ethylene oxide, may be released along with solvents, such as acetone, methanol, dixoane, and methylene chloride in minute quantities. One does not know the extent to which tissue enzymes may be involved in degradation, especially during the latter stages of the process. Researchers have reported that degradation proceeds faster in the center of the PLLA sample than at the surface.[4] The mechanism behind the tissue response to PLLA has not been elucidated. Encapsulation of PLLA leads to collagen deposition, which takes place as the polymer gets degraded. This response may be due to the immune system reaction to the PLLA itself, with degradation products or impurities remaining from the PLLA synthesis. In the case of injected PLLA for the correction of lipoatrophy, the polymer fragments are very small. The surface area to volume ratio is therefore high, which increases the rate of degradation.[7]

EARLY STUDIES

VEGA Study

Sculptra has been safely used in a variety of orthopedic and maxillofacial applications since the mid-1990s and was approved in Europe in 1999 for the cosmetic correction of scars and wrinkles. The goal of this study was to evaluate the efficacy and safety of facial injections of PLLA in HIV-infected patients with severe facial lipoatrophy. This open-label, single-center, uncontrolled, pilot study followed fifty HIV-infected patients over a ninety-six-week period. Patients received PLLA (New-Fill; Biotech Industries SA, Luxembourg) for six weeks, administered as a set of injections at two-week intervals. At each visit, patients received several injections into and around the deep dermis of the atrophied area in each cheek. The majority (86 percent) of the patients received four to five injection sessions. Before the injections, one vial was reconstituted from sterile dry powder of 0.15 g PLLA suspended in 3–4 mL of water. The amount of PLLA injected depended on the severity of skin depression, but a maximum of 4 mL (one vial) of PLLA was injected into each cheek. Patients were evaluated by clinical examinations, facial ultrasonography, and photographs at screening and weeks 6, 24,

48, 72, and 96. All patients experienced increases in skin thickness in the treatment area. Statistically significant increases above baseline values of mean skin thickness were noted at all time points. The increases in mean skin thickness changes above baseline persisted for up to two years. The benefit of PLLA in the correction of facial lipoatrophy in HIV-infected patients was clearly demonstrated, with an evident aesthetic and quality-of-life improvement.[7]

Chelsea and Westminster Study

The objective of this study was to compare immediate versus delayed treatment with Sculptra by injecting it into the dermis overlying the buccal fat pads of HIV-positive persons with facial lipoatrophy receiving antiretroviral therapy. This design was intended to evaluate the temporal association between treatment and improvement in the subjective and objective outcomes. This was a twenty-four-week, open-label, single-center, uncontrolled study in thirty HIV-positive patients with facial lipoatrophy. Individuals were randomized to immediate (at weeks 0, 2, and 4) or delayed (at weeks 12, 14, and 16) injections of PLLA. All patients received a fixed treatment regimen of three injection sessions conducted at two-week intervals. Assessments were based on facial ultrasound, visual analogue scales, the Hospital Anxiety and Depressions Scale (HADS), and taking photographs at weeks 0, 12, and 24. Each vial of Sculptra was reconstituted with 2 mL sterile water for injection and 1 mL 2 percent lidocaine to give a total volume of 3 mL. Up to 3 mL of the reconstituted product was injected bilaterally into multiple points of the cheek and nasolabial areas. Patient visual analogue assessments, photographic assessments, and anxiety and depression scores improved with treatment. Benefits on visual analogue and HADS scores persisted until week 24. The PLLA injections led to improvements in patient self-perception, anxiety, and depression scores in individuals with facial lipoatrophy. Significant changes in mean skin thickness were observed in the areas treated with Sculptra in all patients. A mean increase in skin thickness of approximately 4–6 mm was observed twelve weeks after the initiation of treatment for all patients. There were no differences established among groups at week 24, indicating the treatment was effective regardless of initiating treatment immediately or delaying treatment. It was determined that the benefits of PLLA persisted for at least eighteen weeks beyond the last treatment session.[8]

Blue Pacific Study

The objectives of the Blue Pacific study were to evaluate the quantifiable improvement in lipoatrophy after several deep dermal/subcutaneous injections of PLLA and to evaluate the safety of PLLA usage in repeated treatments in patients with HIV/AIDS. This study also looked into evaluating the long-term durability of the increase in skin thickness, the immediate and long-term patient acceptance of serial treatments of PLLA, and psychological impact of treatment of HIV-associated lipoatrophy with PLLA injections. This was a single-site, open-label study design where ninety-nine patients were enrolled, the majority being Caucasian males. Patients received injections of PLLA into targeted treatment areas. Patients were treated with Sculptra injections scheduled three weeks apart. To assess the correction during the study period and after the last treatment sessions, buccal skin thickness, as well as other study parameters such as photography and caliper skin thickness, was measured. At the end of the treatment, patients exhibited a mean increase of skin thickness of 65.1 percent compared with baseline values. This correction was maintained throughout the twelve-month follow-up period (68.8 percent at six months and 73 percent at twelve months). On a scale of 1–5,

patient satisfaction was 4.5 at the end of the treatment and increased to 4.8 at the twelve-month follow-up. This study reinforces previous studies that PLLA is a safe and effective treatment for HIV-associated facial lipoatrophy. The psychological benefits of treatment were clinically significant, yet the cost and access issues remain for patients who suffer with this condition.[9]

APEX002 Study

This open-label, single-center study evaluated the safety and efficacy of PLLA in patients with facial lipoatrophy. Ninety-nine patients with lipoatrophy were enrolled in the study where they attended one to six treatment sessions at four- to six-week intervals. The majority of patients in the study received three to four treatments as determined by the study physician. The treatment efficacy was monitored by patient and investigator satisfaction while evaluating photographs of patients before each treatment session and at follow-up visits. In the APEX002 study, patients and physicians both rated the degree of lipoatrophy on a scale of 1–5, where 1 was mild and 5 was severe.

Patients rated their level of satisfaction with the outcome of the treatment on a scale of 1–5 (5 being very satisfied, 1 being dissatisfied) where at the final treatment session, the average score was 4.71. Six and twelve months posttreatment, satisfaction levels remained high at 4.74 and 4.75, respectively.

In all of the studies, swelling and/or bruising and edema were reported as treatment-related adverse events. Discomfort during treatment was reported during all the studies except the VEGA study. Postinjection erythema was reported in the Chelsea and Westminster and Blue Pacific studies. Hematoma and inflammation were reported in the VEGA and Chelsea and Westminster studies. In all studies, patients experienced the formation of small, subcutaneous papules (SPs), which were invisible and nonbothersome. In the VEGA study, 44 percent of patients developed SPs, but in 27 percent of those patients, the SPs had disappeared at week 96. Thirty-one percent of patients in the Chelsea and Westminster study developed SPs. Six were in the immediate treatment group and the remainder were in the delayed treatment group. In the APEX002 study, 6 percent of subjects developed SPs, whereas 12 percent of the patients involved in the Blue Pacific study reported having SPs.[9] Although the effects of PLLA have been shown to persist beyond two years, they are not permanent, and so the treatment may need to be repeated to suit the patient's needs. PLLA does not restore lost fat mass at the site of injection but rather expands dermal thickness, predominately through an initial increase in fibroblasts and subsequently an increase in the deposition of collagen fibers. By using PLLA, this may have the advantage that as the underlying mechanism for the lipoatrophy is not clear and is likely to remain in progress in these individuals, the new tissue will not then be lost in the ongoing process of lipoatrophy.[8]

PROCEDURE

As a result of the clinical trials with PLLA, a more standardized procedure has been developed in both the medical and the cosmetic fields. The extent of changes due to facial lipoatrophy demands a global approach to restoration rather than filling a few individual wrinkles. Restoration of soft tissue volume and contours must be accomplished to more closely approximate the youthful, healthy appearance sought by patients. An organized way to proceed with an assessment is to divide the face into three distinct regions: the upper, lower, and midfacial regions. In addition, the face must be assessed in terms of volume, concavities, convexities, and the general quality of the tissue.[2] A large majority of patients with lipoatrophy tend to receive at least

one vial per cheek, whereas a cosmetic patient usually tends to need less.[1–5]

Pretreatment

Unlike some collagen-based fillers, PLLA does not require a skin test before treatment because it is made out of synthetic material. For the reduction of pain during injection, it is optimal to utilize a local anesthetic. One topical anesthetic that gives good results is lidocaine. A mixture of benzocaine, lidocaine, and tetracaine is less likely used as it can trigger a potential allergic contact dermatitis. Nerve blocks can be used when necessary.[5] Addition of 1 cc of 1 percent lidocaine to the vial decreases the need for anesthesia. Some injectors use lidocaine with epinephrine, suggesting they see less of the needle inserts postinjection.

Reconstitution and Dilution

For reconstitution of a uniform homogeneous hydrogel suspension, add 5 mL sterile water twenty-four hours before injection (Figure 10.1). Recently, the use of bacteriostatic water for reconstitution has been shown to increase shelf life to one month. For uniform hydration, do not agitate but allow the powder cake to absorb the sterile H_2O slowly overnight. When the water is added, it will take about five minutes for the powder to dissolve. The mixture is then kept overnight for complete hydration. The now reconstituted product is stored at room temperature to achieve proper viscosity for injection.[1] It is fine to swirl, agitate, or shake hard after hydration overnight.[3,5,7–9] The vial is thoroughly agitated before use. It is optional to add 1 mL of 1 percent lidocaine or lidocaine with epinephrine immediately before injection, making it slowly drip through an eighteen-gauge needle. When added too quickly, lidocaine can precipitate the hydrogel suspension, leading to difficulty, such as clogging, while injecting.

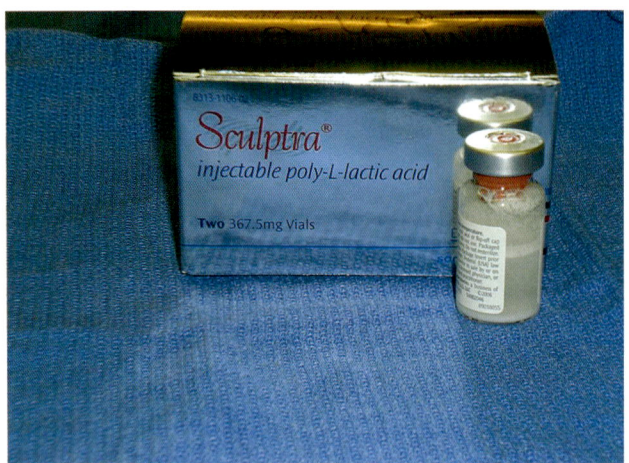

FIG. 10.1.   *For reconstitution of a uniform homogeneous hydrogel suspension, add 5 mL sterile water for injection twenty-four hours before injection.*

To facilitate the withdrawal of PLLA, the eighteen-gauge needle is kept in the vial, allowing equilibration with the atmospheric pressure. Air should not be introduced into the vial on extraction of PLLA because this may also cause precipitation.

Variations in reconstitution volumes exist. Injectors who use regional blocks or local anesthesia may prefer hydration with 6 mL sterile bacteriostatic H_2O alone without the addition of lidocaine. Others may prefer 4 mL sterile bacteriostatic water and 2 mL lidocaine 1 or 2 percent with or without epinephrine. Regardless of the ratio of sterile water to lidocaine, a total reconstitution volume of 6–8 mL per vial provides an optimal suspension for ease of injection and efficacious results. A 6–8 mL dilution may further minimize the possibility of papules or nodules that may occur with more concentrated suspensions of the PLLA hydrogel. The 6–8 mL dilution per vial also provides adequate volume for complete distribution over the lower two-thirds of half the face in cases of severe lipoatrophy. Smaller dilution volumes tend to make uniform distribution and complete coverage more difficult when dealing with larger faces or severe cases.[3,5] An 8–10 cc dilution may be used when injecting near the infraorbital rim. An 8–12 cc dilution is used for the back of the hands, whereas 10 cc provides a volume that results in smooth layering of Sculptra over the hand.

Injection Technique

Sculptra is a product with unique characteristics that make use of this filler different from other currently approved injectable products. There are several basic treatment techniques used when injecting Sculptra into a patient. The tunneling, crosshatch (Figure 10.2A), and fanning techniques (Figure 10.2B) are used in the lower facial regions, and the depot technique is used in the upper part of the face by some injectors. The fanning technique is the most commonly used among injectors. The technique provides fewer injection punctures, resulting in a less painful procedure. It limits bruising, decreases the time of treatment, and decreases the number of needles used. There is a common guideline for administration of Sculptra. The mantra is "treat, wait, assess." It is important to treat correction at each session, to wait for the gradual dermal thickening, and then to assess the need for additional correction after a minimum of four to six weeks.

The suspension of PLLA is injected with a 1-cc Luer-lock syringe with a twenty-five-gauge needle to provide less clogging. More clogging results with the use of a twenty-six-gauge needle. It is important for the injector to assess the viscosity of the suspension before insertion of the needle into the skin to deliver the product. Injection of the material is performed while slowly withdrawing the needle. Most importantly, injection of product must be stopped before withdrawal of the needle so that no product is injected superficially. This will decrease the risk of papule formation. Aspiration through the syringe is performed to prevent injecting into a vessel, which can cause embolization or a skin infarction.[1,5,9,10] PLLA is injected in the deep dermis and subcutaneous junction in one of several injection techniques.

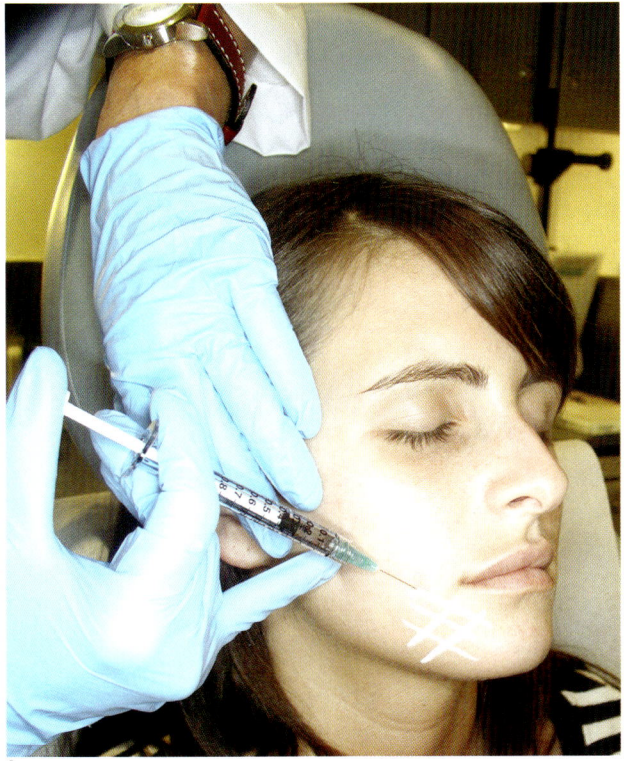

A

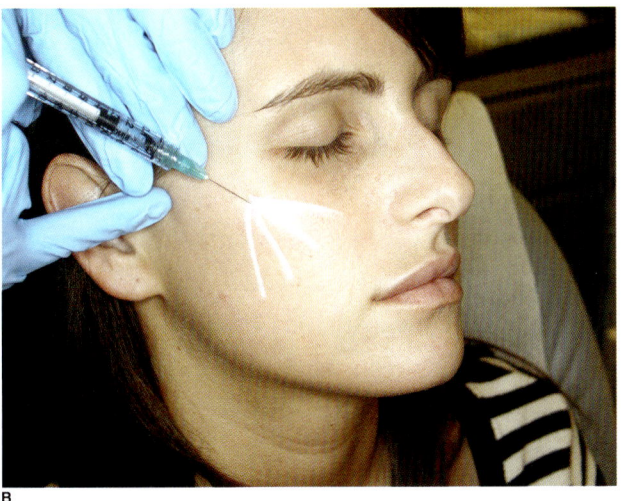

B

FIG. 10.2. *There are several basic treatment techniques used when injecting Sculptra into a patient. The tunneling, crosshatch (A), and fanning techniques (B) are used in the lower facial regions.*

The tunneling technique of 0.1–0.2 mL PLLA delivered at 0.5- to 1-cm intervals was used for FDA approval in the VEGA trial. Using the tunneling technique, the skin is first stretched opposite to the direction of the injection to create a firm

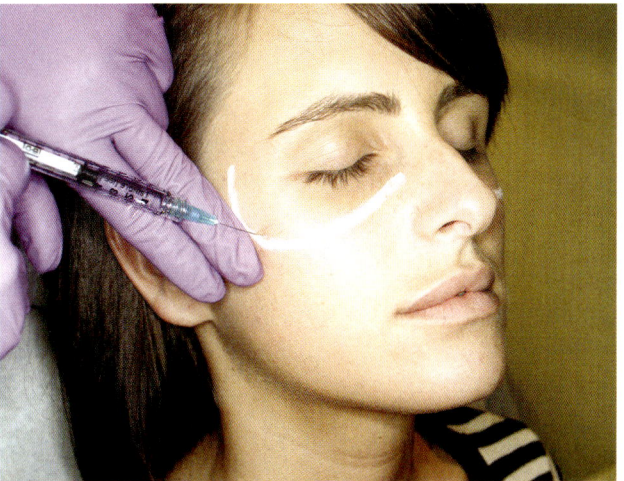

FIG. 10.3. *When using the depot technique in the area of the upper zygoma, Sculptra is injected under the orbicularis oculi muscle, just above the periosteum, in a small bolus dose. A linear threading technique may also be used.*

injection surface. A reflux maneuver should be performed to ensure that a blood vessel has not been entered. By using the tunneling technique in the cheeks or nasolabial area, Sculptra is injected into the deep dermis or subcutaneous layer. A small amount of Sculptra is deposited in the tissue as the needle is withdrawn with a volume of approximately 0.1–0.5 mL of Sculptra per injection depending on the surface area to be injected. The injection site on the skin is gently massaged and the next injection is given adjacent to the site of the previous injection. Multiple injections, which are typically administered in a grid or crosshatch pattern, may be required to cover the targeted area.[5]

When using the depot technique in the area of the upper zygoma, Sculptra is injected under the orbicularis oculi muscle, just above the periosteum, in a small bolus dose. A linear threading technique may also be used (Figure 10.3). Correct injection into the deep dermal space will produce a visible and palpable elevation of the skin at the area of injection. A limited number of injections should be administered into the area with approximately 0.05 mL for each injection. A similar technique is used in the medial temple area, with small injection volumes of approximately 0.05 mL per injection under the superficial fascia at the level of the temporal fascia.[5,6] A linear threading technique may also be used with good results; similarly, the fanning technique may be used in the temple area.

Volume correction of the hands is most commonly performed with a 10 cc dilution using multiple interosseous injections (of approximately 1 cc) tunneled on the back of the hand. However, a bolus injection of 10 cc may be directed under the tenting of the skin on the back of the hand as well. Smooth massage will distribute the Sculptra evenly. Periodic massaging during all treatment sessions may help evenly distribute the product and reduce the risk for papule formation.

Posttreatment

Immediately after the treatment session, cleanse the skin, apply a moisturizer, and thoroughly massage the treated area. Apply an ice pack to the treated area afterward to decrease edema. It is important for the person injecting the patient to massage the treatment area for approximately five minutes to help distribute Sculptra evenly. A nonhomogeneous suspension and incorrect injection of PLLA are significant causes of suboptimal results. Therefore, particular attention should be paid to product reconstitution, level of injection, massaging, and avoidance of overcorrection.[2,6] Although the initial treatment session will provide the patient with an immediate volumizing effect, this is only transient and is a result of the injected sterilized water and injection-associated edema. Cosmetic results will gradually develop several weeks after treatment with desired results typically expected after a series of three to five treatment sessions. Because of the gradual, progressive onset of facial volumizing with injectable PLLA, treatment sessions should be planned at four- to six-

week intervals. This allows the swelling to subside and the lasting effect of injectable PLLA to fully develop before evaluation for further treatment.[2,4–6]

MANAGING PATIENT EXPECTATIONS

It is important that the patient be made fully aware that Sculptra provides a gradual increase in dermal thickness of the treated area with the full effects of the treatment evident in weeks to months. At first, some of the initial injected volume is lost within the first week and the original skin depression may reappear. But the depression should improve within several weeks as the neocollagenesis process of Sculptra occurs. It is often disappointing for patients to watch the initial loss of volume over the first week after treatment and it is essential to make this point clear to the patient.

CURRENT USES AND APPLICATIONS

HIV-Associated Lipodystrophy

Although PLLA has been in use throughout Europe since 1999 for aesthetic purposes, it is currently only approved in the United States for treatment of facial lipoatrophy related to the human immunodeficiency virus (HIV)[11] (Figure 10.4). However, the product has been submitted to the FDA for cosmetic indication and is awaiting approval. The FDA approval was achieved in August 2004. It is unclear as to what factors lead to atrophy in those who suffer from HIV. It may occur as a consequence of the medications normally prescribed for this condition: highly active antiretroviral therapy (HAART), which contains protease inhibitors or nucleotide reverse transcriptase inhibitors.[12] It is estimated that 50 percent of people with HIV who are treated with HAART for more than one year will develop lipoatrophy.[13] It has also been proposed that it results from the actual condition itself.[14] Whatever the cause, the end result is facial

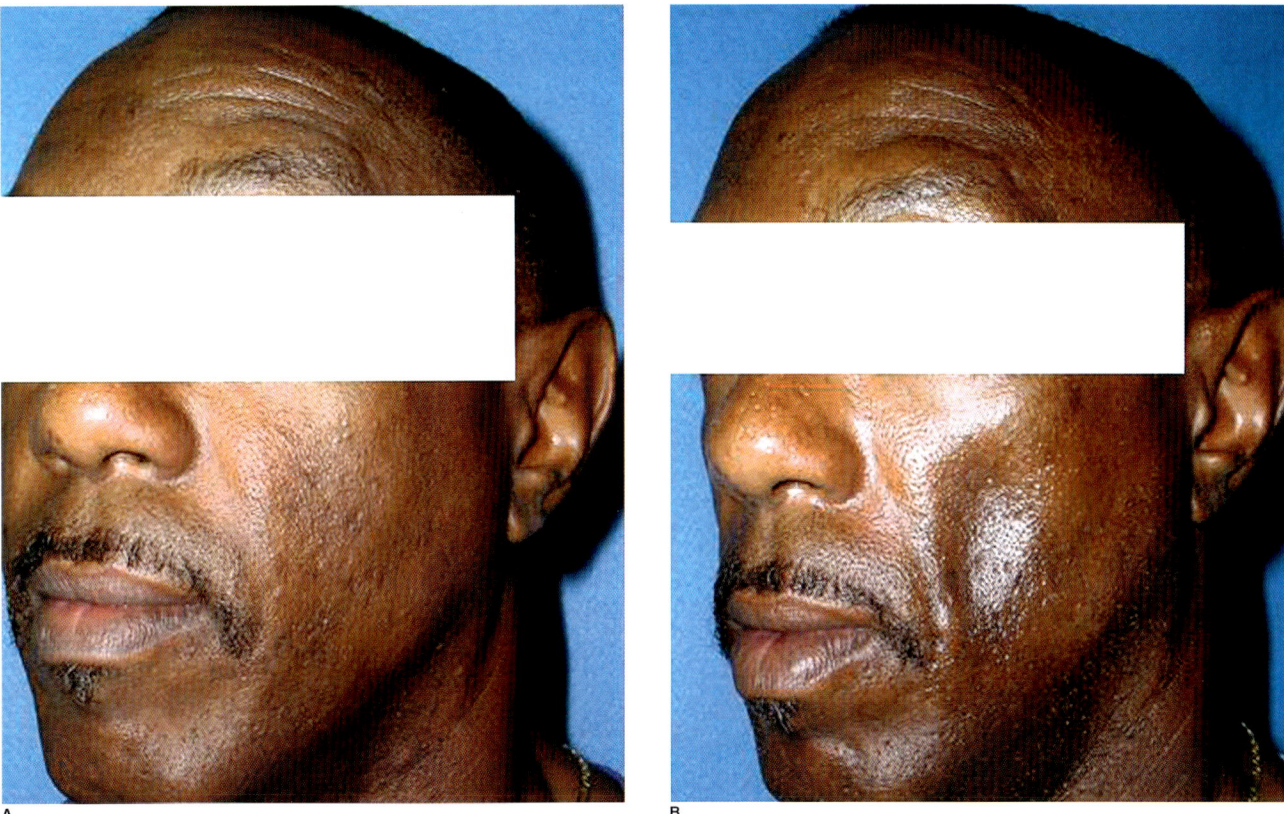

FIG. 10.4. *(A,B) While PLLA has been in use throughout Europe since 1999 for aesthetic purposes, it is currently only approved in the United States for treatment of facial lipoatrophy related to HIV.*

lipoatrophy that can easily be recognized by others. The characteristics of HIV-associated lipodystrophy can have a profound effect on the individual. As treatments for the condition have become more successful, individuals may live longer and have relatively healthy lives. But it is the physical characteristics that may make them stand out. An individual who may otherwise be stable may be clearly identified as suffering from HIV. Lipoatrophy appears in the orbital, buccal, parotid, and preauricular areas. As a result, the area around the eyes looks hollowed out, the cheeks look sunken, and the overall face appears skeletal. For some, this may cause emotional distress as it may signal to onlookers that they have HIV.[15,16]

The redistribution of the fat has major implications for the aesthetic symmetry of the face. The approval of PLLA for use in people who suffer from HIV-related facial lipoatrophy has helped to resolve this issue. A study by Burgess and Quiroga looked at the use of PLLA in treating HIV-associated facial lipoatrophy.[13] All of the enrolled subjects had been previously diagnosed with HIV and had been treated with HAART. All of them were concerned with their physical appearance, specifically the lipoatrophy, which often occurs in such patients. Sixty-one male patients were given multiple treatments (an average of three) over a five-month period. They were monitored for possible adverse reactions. Success was assessed by the patient, physician, and an independent evaluator who was also a physician. At the six-month follow-up, all patients were pleased with the results, as were both physicians. They all rated the results as "excellent" on a scale of 1–4, from "no change" (no improvement) to "excellent" (90–100 percent improvement). Forty-eight patients (79 percent) required three treatment sessions to achieve this result, whereas thirteen patients (21 percent) required four or more treatments. Two subjects developed intradermal papules in the infraorbital region and five developed minor bruising that lasted no more than seven days. There were no allergic or serious adverse reactions.

For these subjects, Sculptra assists in restoring a natural appearance to the face by increasing dermal thickness in areas previously characterized by concavity. The fact that it has been shown to be safe and well tolerated also adds to the advantages of using it in those patients with HIV.

Facial Volume Loss

Facial lipoatrophy is not only seen in people who are suffering from HIV. Other medical conditions such as diabetes, panniculitis, and anorexia nervosa can also result in lipoatrophy and other parts of the body.

Aging, as well, may result in facial lipoatrophy. The factors affecting the aging of the face are a mix of diet, genetics, exposure to the sun, and the simple passage of time. There is often a tendency to see the facial characteristics of old age such as wrinkling and ptosis. As a result, physicians have focused on techniques that reduce superficial lines and wrinkles as well as techniques that tighten the skin. However, aging is characterized by both intrinsic and extrinsic factors that are manifested both on the skin surface and on the subsurface.[17] Collagen loses its elasticity, and gravity pulls the face down. As this happens, the framework of the face begins to sag and degenerate. A concave quality can be seen in the cheeks, temples, preauricular area, and chin. Certain facial areas such as the tear troughs, nasolabial folds, and marionette lines appear deeper than before (Figure 10.5). The resulting sagging can be corrected with surgical

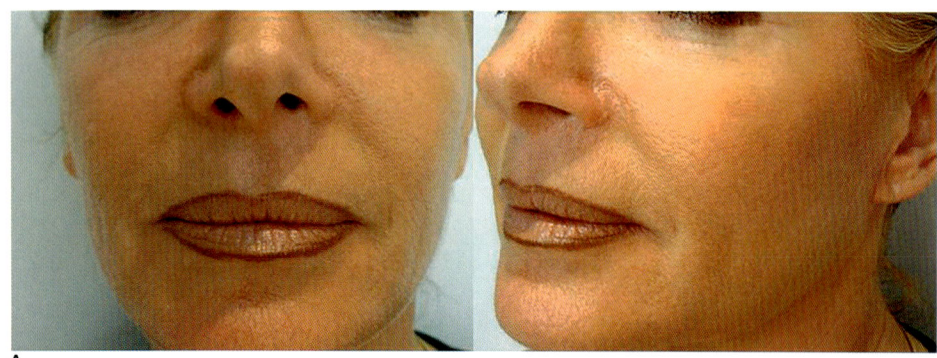

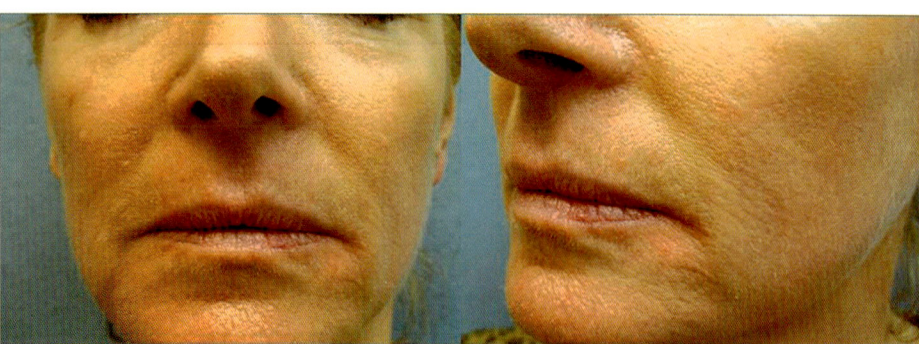

A

B

FIG. 10.5.   (A,B) Certain facial areas such as the tear troughs, nasolabial folds, and marionette lines appear deeper than before.

procedures (such as a face-lift) and laser treatments for tightening, but these procedures do not assist in restoring facial volume loss. Volume loss can be ameliorated with surgical procedures where implants of silicone or polytetrafluoroethylene are inserted. However, these substances remain in the dermis or subcutaneous layer indefinitely. Fat transfer may also be used. This is a more involved procedure as the other invasive procedures are noted for its excessive downtime.

A favorable alternative to these permanent substances is the various fillers now available to treat volume loss. PLLA is often referred to as a sculptor as opposed to a filler. A distinction is made between fillers, which are injectable devices that correct lines and wrinkles, and sculptors, which are injected into the dermis and subcutaneous layers to stimulate collagen production and serve as volumizers.[18] The latter are not utilized for superficial correction.

Sculptors are used as global volumetric fillers that, in the case of PLLA, may last twenty-four months or longer.[3,19] As mentioned previously, the tunneling technique is often used for the lower part of the face and the depot technique is used for the upper region, although linear threading and tunneling may be used with good results in the upper part of the face. It should be stressed that in cases of facial lipoatrophy of any cause, the physician should visualize the face as a three-dimensional plane in receipt of a three-dimensional filler. The concave areas that are being filled must smoothly blend in with the convex areas. The end result should be a face that looks naturally contoured. In the hands of a skilled practitioner, the patient's face will look not only younger and fuller but also natural. It should be kept in mind that PLLA gradually replaces volume over time. The number of necessary treatments is dependent on the level of correction necessary. Treatment sessions should be spaced at least four weeks apart to ensure that overcorrection does not occur.

PLLA in the Hands

As rejuvenation of the facial area has become a standard treatment offered by dermatologists and cosmetic surgeons, it seems natural that the focus should shift to the hands. A patient who wants to look younger by reducing the signs of aging as characterized by volume loss might look for the same effect on their hands. The hands, like the face, reveal one's age through fine lines, wrinkles, photodamage characterized by age spots, and volume loss. Laser and other similar treatments can be used to decrease photodamage, fine lines, and wrinkles. Volumetric fillers, such as PLLA, can be used for volume loss, which will also aid in wrinkle and fine line reduction.[20]

For use in the hands, the product should be reconstituted with 9 mL of sterile bacteriostatic water plus 1 mL of 1 percent lidocaine for each hand. It has been recommended that the linear threading technique be combined with an interosseous approach characterized by tenting of the skin in the treatment area (Figure 10.6). A bolus approach may be used as well, with one injection given under the tented skin and then massaging the area thoroughly. After treatment, the hands should be massaged before

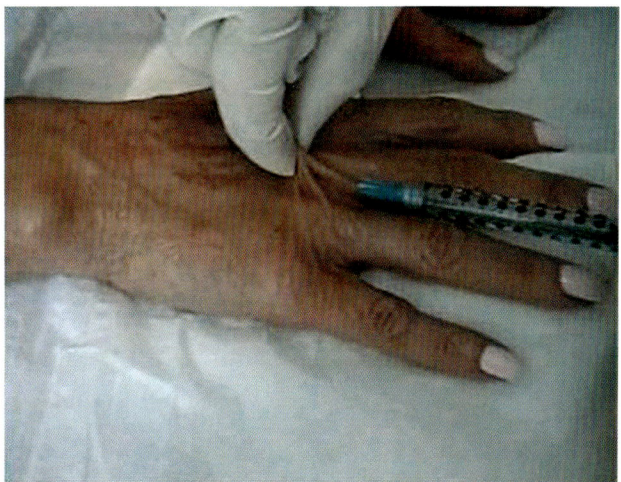

FIG. 10.6. *It has been recommended that the linear threading technique be combined with an interosseous approach characterized by tenting of the skin in the treatment area.*

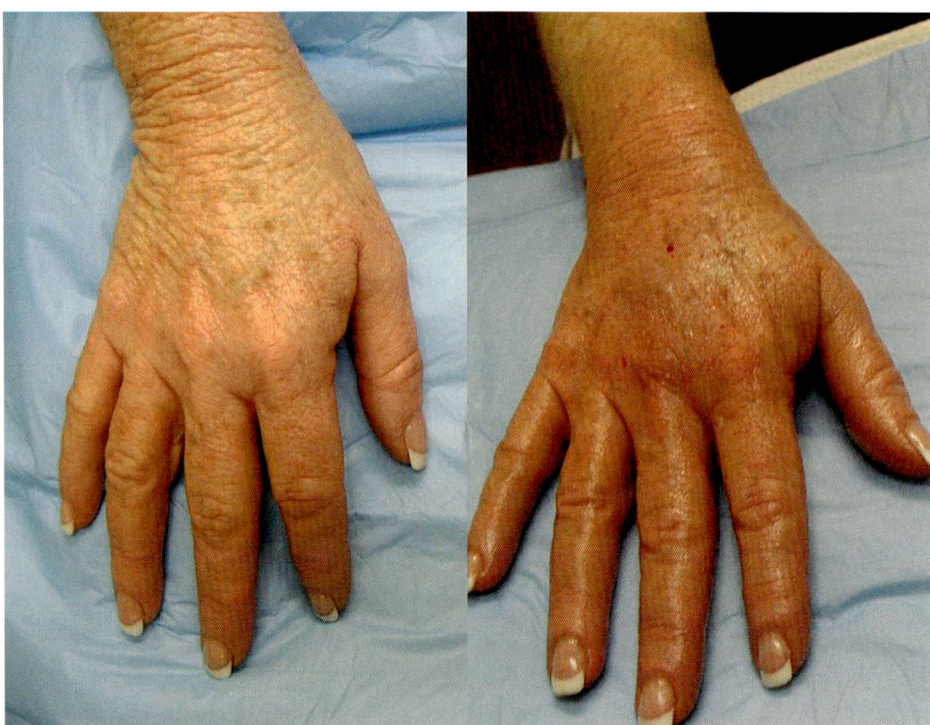

FIG. 10.7.   Patients are also instructed to massage at home for five minutes, five times a day for five days.

application of ice packs. Patients are also instructed to massage at home for five minutes, five times a day for five days (Figure 10.7). As with volume loss in the face, the number of treatments is dependent on the level of correction required by the patient. PLLA may also be used very easily for correction of some surgical deformities or liposuction divots as well.

SAFETY ISSUES

PLLA is a biodegradable compound that has been in use for the past thirty years in devices such as reabsorbable sutures and implants. As such, unlike some other fillers, it is considered safe for use without a skin test. Overall, device-related adverse reactions are rare, and those that do occur do so as a result of incorrect reconstitution, poor injection technique, overcorrection, and deficient injection technique.[21] Thus, it is essential that the injecting physician follow the proper guidelines laid out in the product information provided with each vial of PLLA to avoid these adverse events. Proper techniques and guidelines

are described elsewhere in this chapter. It is important enough to repeat that the injector not overcorrect as is sometimes done with other injectable fillers. The results from PLLA are gradual and progressive and must be tracked over time. Failure to follow these techniques and guidelines may result in SPs, which form from improper dilution of PLLA and improper injection technique[22] (Figure 10.8). These injection-related papules may be prevented with proper dilution, a properly mixed suspension, proper injection depth, and vigorous massage. If papules or nodules form and the patient is distressed, it may be necessary to consider treatment of excision of papules. It should be noted that although these bumps can be palpable to the patients, they are often invisible and nonpathological. A bump resulting from a foreign body reaction will respond to a dilute triamcinolone injection. A bump resulting from clumping of PLLA may require subcision (breaking up) of nodule with an eighteen-gauge needle followed by injection of sterile water to dilute the PLLA and

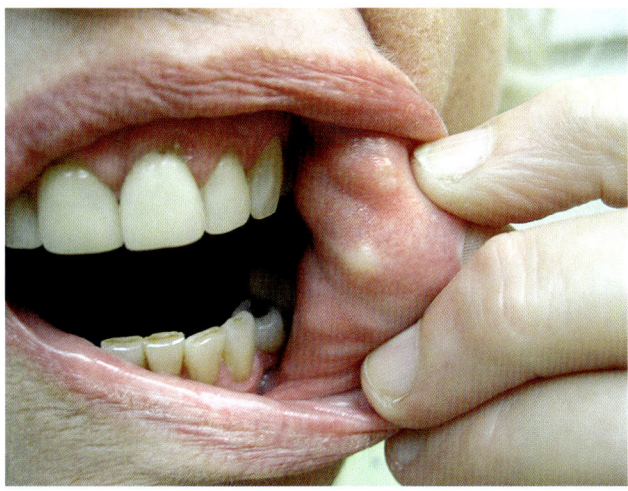

FIG. 10.8. *Failure to follow these techniques and guidelines may result in SPs, which form from improper dilution of PLLA and improper injection technique.*

massage or surgical excision. Granulomas have been noted in the past as with all fillers. Most recently reported were PLLA granulomas in a patient previously injected with silicone. Late-onset granulomas may be treated with triamcinolone, f-fluorouracil, or methylprednisolone. Systemic therapy with low-dose prednisolone, doxycycline, or tetracycline has also been reported.

Additionally, injections into infected or inflamed skin are to be avoided. Patients who are allergic to any ingredients in PLLA should not be treated with the product.

CONCLUSION

Volume loss is a major component of aging. It should not be overlooked when treating patients who seek to "reverse" the signs of aging. Although other treatments and devices concentrate on lines, wrinkles, and age spots, PLLA is a volumetric filler that helps to recontour and sculpt the face. PLLA is a perfect complement to other devices used in rejuvenation. Lasers, fillers, and Botox can be used along with PLLA to ensure the patient's satisfaction. Its importance in treating patients with HIV-associated

lipodystrophy has been proven. Sculptra is a long-lasting but nonpermanent solution to volume loss whatever the cause.

REFERENCES

1. Woerle B, Hanke CW, Satteler G. Poly-L-lactic acid: a temporary filler for soft tissue augmentation. *J Drugs Dermatol*. 2004; **3**(4):385–389.

2. New treatment options in lipoatrophy. *Dermatol Times*. 2005;Suppl:1–16.

3. Sherman RN. Sculptra: the new three-dimensional filler. *Clin Plast Surg*. 2006; **33**(4):539–550.

4. Sculptra package insert.

5. Kronenthal RL. Biodegradable polymers in medicine and surgery. *Polymer Sci Technol*. 1975; **8**:119–137.

6. Dermik Aesthetic, The art and science of Sculptra (injectable poly-L-lactic acid) Slide Kit, September 2004.

7. Hanke CW, Redbord KP. Safety and efficacy of poly-L-lactic acid in HIV lipoatrophy and lipoatrophy of aging. *J Drugs Dermatol*. 2007; **6**:123–128.

8. Valantin MA, Aubron-Olivier C, Chosn J, Laglenne E, Pauchard M, Schoen H, Bousquet R, Katz P, Costagliola D, Katalama C. Polylactic acid implants (New-Fill) to correct facial lipoatrophy in HIV-infected patients: results of the open-label study VEGA. *AIDS*. 2003; **17**:2471–2477.

9. Moyle GJ, Lysakova L, Brown S, Sibtain N, Healy J, Priest C, Mandalia S, Barton SE. A randomized open-label study of immediate versus delayed polylactic acid injections for the cosmetic management of facial lipoatrophy in persons with HIV infection. *HIV Med*. 2004; **5**:82–87.

10. Enghard P, Humble G, Mest D. Safety of Sculptra: a review of clinical trial data. *J Cosmet Laser Ther*. 2005; **7**(3):201–205.

11. Barton SE, Englehard P, Conant M. Poly-L-lactic acid for treatment of HIV-associated facial lipoatrophy: a review of the clinical studies. *Int J STD AIDS*. 2006; **17**:429–435.

12. Lam SM, Azzizzadeh B, Graivier M. Injectable poly-L-lactic acid (Sculptra): technical considerations in soft-tissue contouring. *Plast Reconstr Surg*. 2006;Suppl **1**:55S–63S.

13. Burgess CM, Quiroga RM. Assessment of the safety and efficacy of poly-L-lactic acid for the treatment of HIV-associated facial lipoatrophy. *J Am Acad Dermatol.* 2005; **52**:233–239.

14. Carr A, Samaras K, Thorisdottir A. Diagnosis, prediction and natural occurrence of HIV-1 protease-inhibitor-associated lipodystrophy, hyperlipidemia and diabetes mellitus: a cohort study. *Lancet.* 1999; **353**:2093–2099.

15. Garcia-Viejo MA, Ruiz M, Martinez E. Strategies for treating HIV-related lipodystrophy. *Expert Opin Invest Drugs.* 2001; **10**:1443–1456.

16. O'Donovan CA, Hourihan M, Petrak J, et al., Psycho-social adjustment to facial lipoatrophy in people with HIV. Presented at the 7th International Workshop on Adverse Drug Reactions and Lipodystrophy in HIV. Dublin, Ireland, November 13–16, 2005. Abstract 34. *Antiviral Ther.* 2005; **10**:L24.

17. James J, Carruthers A, Carruthers J. HIV-associated facial lipoatrophy. *Dermatol Surg.* 2002; **28**:979–986.

18. Lowe NJ. Introductory comment. *J Eur Acad Dermatol Venereol.* 2006; **20**:1.

19. Weinkle S. Facial assessments: identifying the suitable pathway to facial rejuvenation. *J Eur Acad Dermatol Venereol.* 2006; **20**:7–11.

20. Thioly-Bensoussan D. A new option for volumetric restoration: poly-L-lactic acid. *J Eur Acad Dermatol Venereol.* 2006; **20**:12–16.

21. Lowe NJ. Dispelling the myth: appropriate use of poly-L-lactic acid and clinical consideration. *J Eur Acad Dermatol Venereol.* 2006; s**1**:2–6.

22. Sadick NS, Burgess C. Clinical experience of adverse outcomes associated with poly-L-lactic acid. *J Drugs Dermatol.* In press.

Chapter 11

LIPO TRANSFER

by

Lisa M. Donofrio, MD

For volumizing the aging face, few fillers display the versatility, endurance, and safety profile as autologous fat. Fat is the perfect choice for those patients wishing to add contour and projection to an otherwise flat visage. Understanding the concepts of facial volumetric aging is paramount to success with any filler but especially one as long lasting as autologous fat. In youth, facial contours are "balanced" with fat resplendent and diffuse. As the face ages, the fat becomes "unbalanced" and dependent on its overall body content. Recent anatomical research suggests that the face is made up of discrete separate fat compartments and that these compartments age individually.[1] This is perfectly illustrated by comparing the atrophic aging seen all over in a patient of ascetic body type with the combination of hypertrophic and atrophic aging seen in a more corpulent individual. It appears that increasing body fat leads to deposits or hypertrophy of fat in certain fat compartments, while others remain atrophic (Figure 11.1A,B). It is unknown as to why the face ages compartmentally, but luckily, the transfer of autologous fat back into the atrophic areas can restore a sense of balance and youth to the face.

PLANNING

During the initial consult, it is helpful for patients to bring in a photograph of what they looked like ten years ago. It is important to ask the weight of the patient currently as compared with the time of the old photograph. This gleans useful information when planning the amount of volume necessary to rebalance the facial fat compartments. The initial consult is also a good time to gather information on the expectations of the patient. Although oftentimes dramatic tightening can be seen by subcutaneous filling with resultant skin redraping, filling should be reserved for those patients who desire contour changes and not solely tight skin. In particular, laxity of the neck often warrants discussion of traditional surgical-lifting procedures oftentimes in combination with autologous fat filling. Contraindications to the fat transfer procedure include coagulation disorders (natural and iatrogenic), disorders of lipid metabolism, severe chronic disease states, acute infection, or organ failure. History of deep vein thrombosis or pulmonary embolus or HIV-infected patients on current HAART warrants individual case-by-case consideration. Although somewhat obvious, a very thin patient

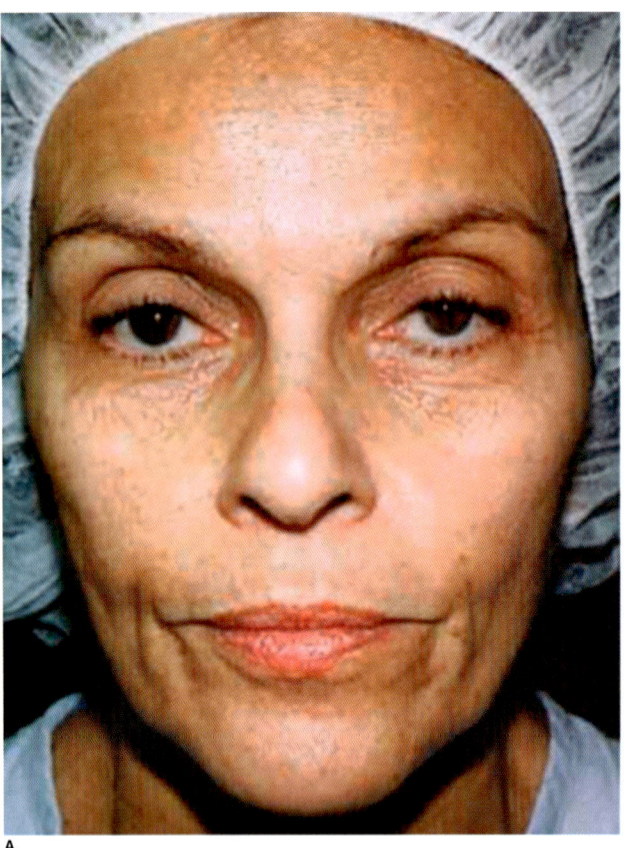
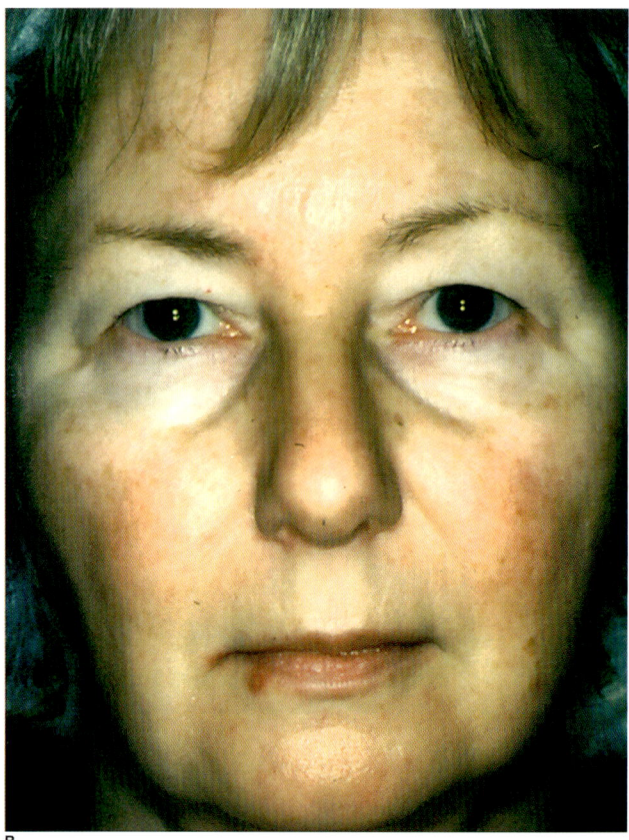
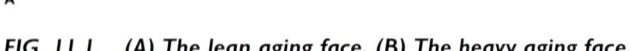

FIG. 11.1.   (A) The lean aging face. (B) The heavy aging face.

may not have a "donor" site to harvest the fat from and would be a better candidate for "off-the-shelf" fillers.

PREOPERATIVE

Assessing and documenting the health of the patient should be done before the procedure by evaluating laboratory blood values. On the day of the procedure, it is advisable to submit an in-office pregnancy test for all females of childbearing potential. Premedication with cephalexin begins the day before the original harvesting (liposuction) procedure and continues for six days after. Erythromycin or ciprofloxacin may alternatively be used in penicillin-allergic patients. A mild anxiolytic such as diazepam 5 mg p.o. is offered to anxious patients half an hour before the procedure. The donor site on the body is

selected from an area that will ultimately benefit the patient cosmetically. Both the donor area and the face are cleansed with antimicrobial soap. The donor area is delineated with a surgical marker as are the areas requiring fat transplantation on the face. It is helpful at this point to make notes of estimated transplant volumes, baseline asymmetries, and bony landmarks.

FAT HARVESTING

The patient is placed on a sterile operating table cover and draped with sterile sheets. Klein tumescent fluid is infiltrated into the donor site either manually or with the assistance of an infiltration pump until the end point of tissue turgidity is reached (Table 11.1). Fat extraction takes place with manual suction only by attaching a 10-ml luer lock syringe

TABLE 11.1. Tumescent Formula Employed for Lipo transfer

Klein tumescent fluid
Normal saline 1 l
Xylocaine 1% 50 ml
Epinephrine 1 mg
Sodium bicarbonate 12.5 meq

onto an open-tipped extraction cannula. The plunger is pulled back as the cannula is moved through the adipose tissue in a back and forth motion. After filling the syringe, a cap is fixed and the syringe centrifuged at 3,400 rpm for ten to twenty seconds. The infranate composed of blood and tumescent fluid is decanted and the spun fat transferred to 1-ml syringes before injection into the face. After the fat extraction, the donor site is dressed with an absorbable dressing, and a light compression garment is applied for three days.

GENERAL TRANSPLANTATION TECHNIQUE

Fat is always transferred to the face with a blunt eighteen- to twenty-gauge cannula attached to a 1-ml syringe. Entry sites are made with an eighteen-gauge needle. Fat is deposited in all layers of tissue when possible, taking advantage of multiple incision sites to fully sculpt the treatment areas. Small aliquots of fat are deposited on the withdrawal phase of the cannula stroke. Occasionally, pearls or droplets are placed. Passes should deposit less than 0.1 ml of fat. Even pressure is applied on the injection cannula by using the palm of the dominant hand on the plunger. Care is taken to avoid placing too much fat in any one area.

Specific Transplantation Technique by Area

Forehead and Temple

A young person's forehead is convex in its anterior dimension and the temples are full extending beyond the line of the lateral brow. With aging, the forehead flattens and temples become hollow resulting in a downward displacement of skin and brow ptosis.

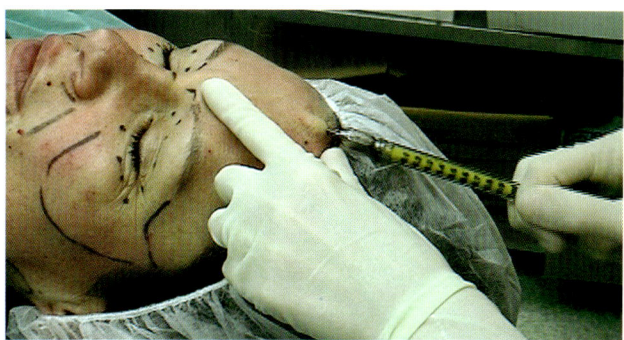

FIG. 11.2. *Forehead augmentation.*

The goal of forehead augmentation is to arc the soft tissues away from the calvarium, thus lifting the brow. The brow can be filled directly as well, and this will be covered in depth later. Forehead augmentation takes place in the deep subcutaneous/muscular plane. Fat should not be placed subgaleal since this is an avascular plane and will not support the sustenance of fat. The deep subcutaneous plane of the forehead is dense and fibrous. Fat placement is arduous and oftentimes prone to irregularities and prolonged edema. Judicious placement of small linear threads of fat at incision sites perpendicular to the brow, parallel with the fibers of the frontalis, is recommended. Prior administration of botulinum toxin to the frontalis muscle lends immobility to the area and may lessen the chance of movement associated with clumping of the fat. Augmentation volumes can approach 10 ml when the entire forehead is addressed (Figure 11.2).

The temporal extension of the buccal fat pad atrophies with age. Gaunt hollow temples are pathognomonic for both aging and disease states. Fat when replaced in the temples has the ability to lift the lateral third of the brow, widen the upper third of the face, and bestow an aesthetic appearance of health and vitality. Augmentation of the temple is approached through an incision at the superiormost portion of the temporal fossa. A curved cannula is especially helpful here allowing the placement of fat deep to the temporalis muscle. Each temple can easily be augmented with 3–5 ml of fat (Figure 11.3).

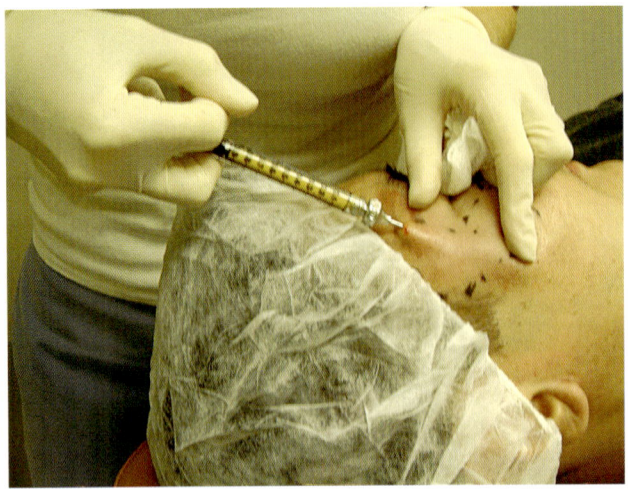

FIG. 11.3.   Temple augmentation.

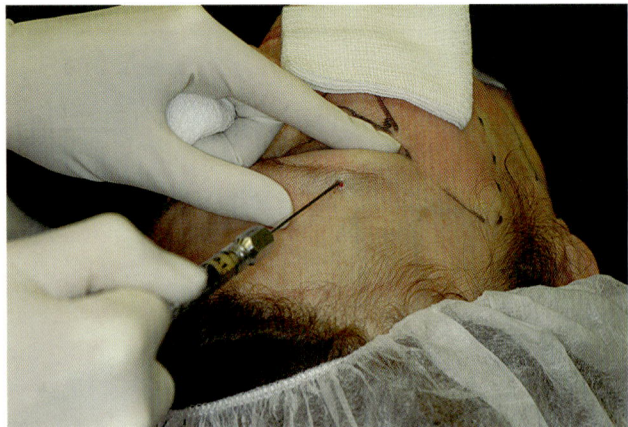

FIG. 11.4.   Brow augmentation.

Brow

A youthful brow is full. As the face ages, the orbital rim becomes unmasked and the eye appears proptotic with more lid shown than in youth. Persistence of the medial upper lid fat and a peaking of the medial lid due to fat loss in this area are common. The goals of lid augmentation are to drop the lid crease and to arc the brow anteriorly and superiorly, thus lifting the skin of the lid. Brow augmentation is most predictable when approached from incision sites along the brow. Fat is deposited to the lid crease as a "droplet" of less than 0.1 ml and the "tail" of the droplet pulled superiorly. This is injected under the orbicularis oculi muscle anterior to the superior orbital septum (Figure 11.4).

Suborbital

There are two types of suborbital aging: atrophic and hypertrophic. Atrophic suborbital aging occurs with loss of volume from the inferior orbital ridge to the lower tarsus. Oftentimes, there is a demarcation of the orbit and a hollowing under the eyes. Due to loss of subcutaneous fat in the suborbital area and dermal thinning, the orbicularis oculi is readily visible under the skin leading to a purple discoloration. This in combination with the inferiorly cast shadow caused by the globe leads to the appearance of dark circles. Hypertrophic suborbital aging is when the suborbital area is full and the fat is anteriorly placed in relation to the upper cheek mass. There is very often a trough along the dermal insertion of the orbital septum. In both cases, there is an interruption of the eye–cheek continuum. Suborbital fat infiltration takes place in the suborbicularis plane. From an inferiorly based incision in the central cheek or in the nasolabial fold, fat is placed in droplets along the orbital rim, moving from medial to lateral. A second incision in the mid-lateral cheek affords easy access to the lateral suborbital area and malar platform. Horizontal placement of fat from the lateral canthus should not be attempted nor should superficial placement due to the risk of lumps and ridging. When treating atrophic suborbital aging, fat augmentation occurs in the direct suborbital area from the orbital rim to the tarsus. Treating just the cheek in these individuals can accentuate the hollows. This is in contrast to hypertrophic variant of suborbital aging where the superior cheek is addressed up to and including the tear trough, but the immediate suborbital area is avoided. Suborbital filling should be conservative with volumes not exceeding 2 ml per side. Care should be taken to blend and feather the edges and to place minute amounts with each pass (Figure 11.5).

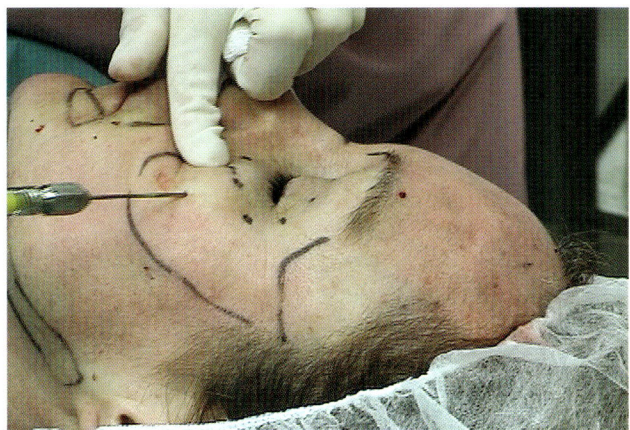

FIG. 11.5. Suborbital augmentation.

Cheek

The cheek really comprises three areas: the central malar area or cheek "apple," the lateral zygoma, and the buccal hollow. Most often, augmentation takes place in all three contiguous areas, blending and feathering the edges. However, certain aesthetic circumstances may warrant filling only one or two of these areas. For instance, in the case of malar hypoplasia where the goal is to advance the midface, the buccal and zygomatic areas may be left alone, or in the case of a round cherubic face, only the lateral zygoma may be treated to establish contour. The cheek is routinely the most predictable area for "take" of autologous fat. Desiring cheek volume or cheek projection is the primary reason for choosing autologous fat over other nonautologous small volume fillers. It is also a wonderful area for the novice fat transplant surgeon to get started. The goal of cheek augmentation in the central malar area is to project the face forward, thus suspending and lifting the lower face. Fat is best placed around the zygomaticus muscle as well as in the subcutaneous fat via an incision lateral to or in the nasolabial fold. The central malar area can hold 5–7 ml of fat deposited as "threads." Oftentimes, a second incision lateral to the zygomatic arch is useful to crosshatch the area and deposit the optimal amount of fat in the deep central

cheek. This incision can also be used for zygomatic enhancement. The buccal hollows in some individuals when deep can lead to a gaunt or sickly look. Fat replacement in this area makes the face appear younger as well as healthier. The buccal area contains tough fibrous tissue, so transplantation of fat at this anatomic site can be arduous. It is very important that fat be threaded in small aliquots with care taken to crosshatch and fan. In addition, the lateralmost aspect must be blended past the parotid fusion line to prevent an apparent "bunching" of tissue on smiling. The buccal hollows commonly take 3–5 ml of fat.

Lateral Face

To avoid a central chubby cheek or juvenile appearance, the lateral face must be addressed for balance. This includes the temporal fossa as well as the face anterior to the ear up to the buccal hollow. For elucidation of this area, have the patient lie down. There will be a sharp demarcation along the investment of the parotid fascia and a relative drop-off in volume as compared to the midface. This area can be delineated in marker at this time. Like the buccal area, the lateral face is resplendent in tough fibrous tissue. The lateral face not including the temple can hold at least 5 ml of fat and in some situations 10 ml per side.

Mandible and Chin

The mandibular angle, like the lateral third of the cheek, balances out any fullness in the medial third of the face. Augmentation of the jawline takes place not only in the anterior plane but also in the inferior plane. Fat in a young face wraps around the jawline, blunting the mandibulo-cervical angle. As the face ages, the definition between the mandible and the neck gets obscured. This creates not only a static diminution of the prominence of the mandible but also an accentuation of positional laxity. The mandible is approached through multiple incisions perpendicular to its border. Fat is infiltrated from an

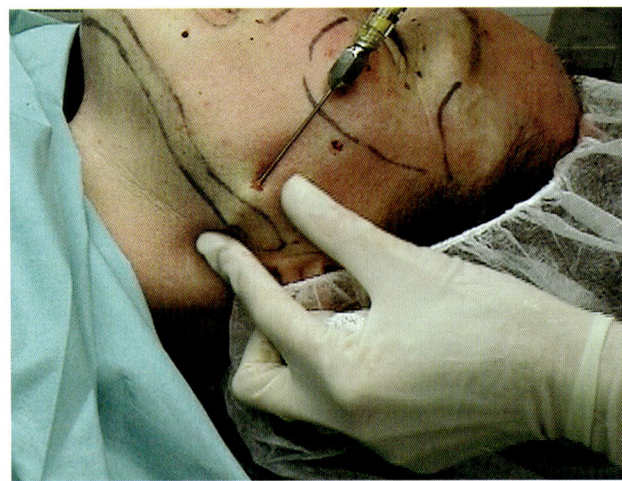

FIG. 11.6. Mandible augmentation.

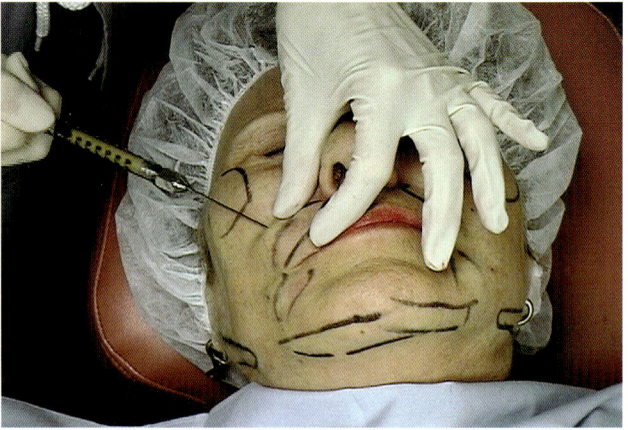

FIG. 11.7. Nasolabial fold augmentation.

incision site approximately 1 cm above the angle of the mandible fanning laterally and inferiorly so the fat ends 1 cm below the angle on the superior portion of the neck (Figure 11.6). This serves to not only define the jawline but also "borrow" skin from the neck, thus lifting the neck. In addition, the superior portion of the neck is cast in the shadow of the mandible and visually recedes. The augmentation can be carried as far medially as the chin where fat is placed in the prejowl sulcus and the submental area forming a "sling." This serves to alleviate the isolation of the chin seen with aging as well as lifting the chin anteriorly. If more chin projection is desired, the mentum itself can be augmented moving from a lateral incision, threading fat toward the midline. The jawline and chin can take upward of 20 ml of autologous fat.

Nasolabial Fold

Rarely should the nasolabial fold solely be addressed with fat. Due to the robustness of fat as a filler and its tendency for permanence, nasolabial fold filling alone can leave the patient looking simian. Rather, the fold should be addressed as a contiguous unit to the cheek and the prementum. Fat should be placed perpendicular to the fold, coming from an incision lateral to the fold, traversing the crease itself. The augmentation can be carried as far medial as the philtrum being

careful to pull threads of fat across the fold. Fat is almost never placed directly into the fold in a parallel direction since this only serves to relocate the fold medially (Figure 11.7). The labiomental crease being similar in structure should be addressed likewise. Fat should be placed across the crease and in doing so will subcise the retaining ligaments in this area. If desired, from the same incision, the prejowl sulcus can be reached. Again, the labiomental crease is not a discrete structure and its relation to the neighboring buccal cheek area should be addressed. Typically, the nasolabial fold and the labiomental crease each takes 1–2 ml of fat per side.

Lips

Lip augmentation with fat is rarely a permanent event. Due to the bulky nature of fat, swelling is often prolonged and the aesthetic outcome unrefined. However, if fat is desired for augmentation of the lips, it is best administered from an incision lateral to the nasolabial fold for the top lip and lateral to the labiomental crease for the bottom lip. Fat is placed in droplets close to the mucosa, staying perpendicular to the vermilion. This approach has the best chance for lip eversion (Figure 11.8). Understanding lip proportion and aesthetics is paramount to a successful outcome. The upper lip comprises a

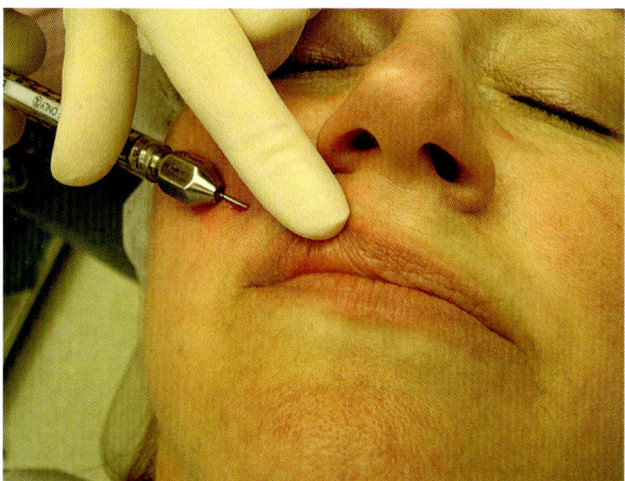

FIG 11.8.   Lip augmentation.

medial tubercle and two lateral prominences. The lower lip contains two discrete balls with a cleft coursing centrally. Judicious placement in this pattern is most likely to result in a visually pleasing, natural lip. The upper and lower lips usually take 1 ml of fat per side. To attenuate vertical lip rhytids, fat can be placed perpendicular to the vermilion along the direction of the orbicularis oris muscle. The same incision lateral to the nasolabial fold can be used. Fat is placed on the immediate subdermal plane, above the muscle. The entire prementum is treated routinely with 1 ml of fat per side.

Hands

Atrophic changes in the dorsum of the hand lead to an unmasking of the vessels and extensor tendons. Filling the hand up with fat softens the contours and covers the sinuous changes. From a single incision on the dorsal wrist, the cannula is threaded toward the intertendinous spaces. Four bolus injections of 1–2 ml fat each are given.

After the cannula is withdrawn, the hand is massaged and the fat kneaded diffusely. Extra fat is placed where incomplete filling has occurred, and new incision sites used if needed to facilitate distribution of the fat.

POSTOPERATIVE CARE

An elastic garment is worn by the patient on the liposuction site for twenty-four hours or longer if dictated for comfort. Frequently, absorbent dressings are applied under the garment to wick the drainage of tumescent fluid. Patients are routinely given an intramuscular steroid to lessen swelling such as triamcinolone acetonide 20 mg as well as the herbal supplement arnica montana p.o. Ice is applied for ten minutes out of every hour for the first twenty-four hours while the patient is awake. The patient is instructed to avoid water submersion like swimming or tub bathing until all incision sites on the face and body have healed. Swim goggles are also to be avoided for the first few weeks as are inversion exercises due to the increase in periorbital edema that both of these can incur.

SIDE EFFECTS

Rare documented side effects include middle cerebral artery infarction, skin necrosis, and blindness.[2–5] However, side effects historically documented in the literature are very different from those seen in actuality with a microinjection pressure blunt cannula technique. Due to the inability of a blunt cannula to canalize a vessel, and the low pressure incurred by injection via a 1-ml syringe, vascular occlusive events should never be seen. Rare side effects include infection, overcorrection, asymmetries, lumps, injection site tattoos, and/or dimpling and fat cysts. Common sequella such as ecchymosis or edema can often last two weeks.

FRESH VERSUS FROZEN FAT

Fat works best when deposited in stages. This ensures that each fat transfer is not overcorrected and allows for more control over final volumes and contour. The easiest way for patients is to use their own banked and stored frozen fat. Much controversy exists around the use of frozen fat as a "viable" alternative to fresh fat.

Well-controlled human studies are lacking, and animal studies are difficult to interpret and rife with inconstancies. If using frozen fat, certain guidelines of care should be followed. The triglycerides should be left in the syringe when freezing. The fat should be frozen slowly, if possible in a stepped manner. The vials of fat should be meticulously labeled with such identifying information as the patients' name and social security number and the date of performing the procedure. The fat should be stored in a constant temperature freezer with a temperature-monitoring log and alarm backup. On defrosting for use, the fat should be rapidly thawed to prevent the formation of ice crystals. An easy method is to place the fat-filled syringe inside a surgical glove and have the patient hold it in the axilla, against the skin. Before placing in the face, the fat should be verified by an assistant and the verification initialed in the chart. Since frozen fat sterility has only been documented up to twenty-four months, the standard of care at this time is to freeze the fat for up to two years.[6] The author has found frozen fat to often incur long-term correction when used after an initial fresh fat procedure, but an individual surgeon's experiences with frozen fat will certainly dictate its appropriateness.

LONGEVITY

Many surgeons have documented long-term results utilizing a structural microinjection fat grafting technique.[7–9] The author has found that certain areas of the face tend to retain fat better than others, the

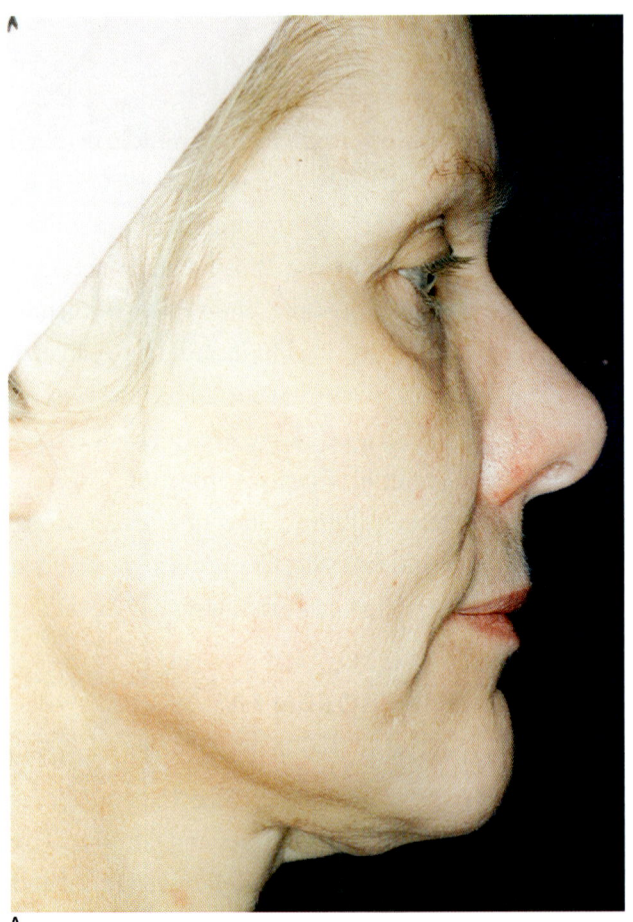
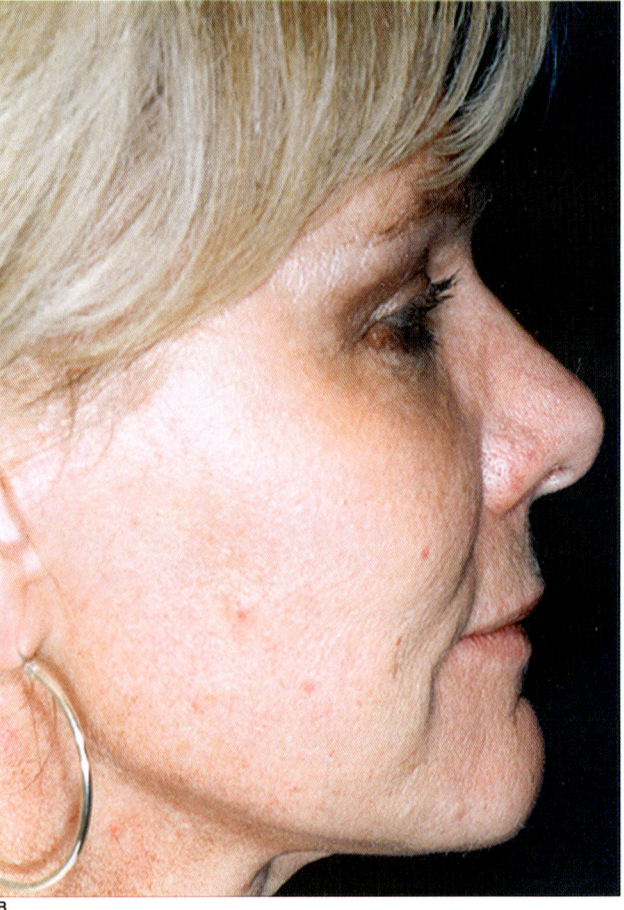

FIG. 11.9.   (A) Before and (B) twenty months after pan-facial fat augmentation.

highest retention areas being the cheeks and periorbital area. Fat appears to achieve the best results where fat atrophy is the problem. This may explain why in the perioral area, where bone remodeling and mucosal atrophy is the cause of the atrophic insult, fat take is poor. Patients desiring further correction in low retention areas are often encouraged to augment with hyaluronic acid or calcium hydroxyl apatite fillers; however, these small volume fillers are not capable of the dramatic tissue shifts achievable with fat augmentation in the structural plane (Figure 11.9A,B).

REFERENCES

1. Rohrich RJ, Pessa JE. The fat compartments of the face: anatomy and clinical implications for cosmetic surgery. *Plastic Reconstructive Surgery* 2007 Jun;**119**(7): 2219–2227.

2. Teimourian B. Blindness following fat injections. *Plastic and Reconstructive Surgery* 1988 **82**: 361.

3. Feinendegen DL, Baumgartner RW, Schroth G, Mattle HP, Tschopp H. Middle cerebral artery occlusion and ocular fat embolism after autologous fat injection in the face. *Journal of Neurology* 1988 **245**: 53–54.

4. Danesh-Meyer HV, Savino PJ, Sergott RC. Case reports and a small case series; ocular and cerebral ischemia following facial injection of autologous fat. *Archives of Opthamology* 2001 **119**: 777–778.

5. Egido JA, Arroyo R, Marcos A, Jimenez-Alfaro I. Middle cerebral artery embolism and unilateral visual loss after autologous fat injection into the glabellar area. *Stroke* 1993 **24**: 615–616.

6. Narins RS. Long-term sterility of fat frozen for up to 24 months. *Journal of Drugs in Dermatology* 2003 Oct;**2**(5): 505–507.

7. Donofrio LM. Panfacial volume restoration with fat. *Dermatologic Surgery* 2005 Nov;**31**(11 Pt 2): 1496–1505.

8. Donofrio LM. Structural lipoaugmentation: a panfacial technique. *Dermatologic Surgery* 2000 Dec;**26**(12): 1129–1134.

9. Coleman SR. Long term results of fat transplants: controlled demonstrations. *Aesthetic Plastic Surgery* 1995 **19**: 421–425.

Chapter 12

BIOALCAMID®

by

David J. Goldberg, MD

INTRODUCTION

A wide variety of synthetic fillers are now available. Such fillers can be divided into a variety of categories. One descriptive category relates to filler duration. Fillers can last in the human body for short periods of time or they can be permanent. BioAlcamid® is a permanent prosthesis-type filler. It is used in many parts of the world but is not yet available in the United States. An ideal biomaterial must be nonallergic, inert, sterile nonpyogenic, noncancer producing, stable, incapable of migrating, and most importantly biologically compatible with the host tissue. The latter factor is required because it impacts on the ability of the filler to coexist with surrounding tissues without either stimulating the immune system or causing persistent inflammatory reactions.

BIOALCAMID®

BioAlcamid®, a synthetic polyalkylamide manufactured by Polymekon in Italy, is a permanent implant that fulfills some, but certainly not all, of the aforementioned requirements.

CLINICAL STUDIES

There are only a few studies that have evaluated the safety and efficacy of BioAlcamid® implants.[1-6] In a clinical study performed by Protopapa et al., eighty BioAlcamid® implants were injected into seventy-three subjects aged sixteen to forty-eight years (forty females and thirty-three males).[1] All patients were HIV+ and suffered from lipodystrophy syndrome to varying degrees. Individuals with uncompromised diabetes mellitus and psychiatric disorders and pregnant women were excluded from the study. No prior skin tests were done. Initial implants were placed in the face. Ultimately, three patients requested further corrections to their buttocks; four patients requested corrections to their limbs. The BioAlcamid® was injected into the subcutaneous layer.

Those with facial deformities received up to 35 ml of the product; correction of buttock deficits required up to 1,600 ml of the biopolymer. In over 90 percent of cases, a second injection of BioAlcamid® was given four weeks after the first injection to optimize implant appearance. Nineteen-gauge needles were used to inject the material into the face; sixteen-gauge needles were used in the buttocks and legs. Not more than 15 ml was injected at any one site. Multiple injections were administered until total correction of the deficit was obtained. All patients were given antibiotics after injection of the prosthesis.

All patients were evaluated at four weeks, two months, and one year after implantation. Three patients were followed up for three years. Immediately after injection, the material appeared soft. Postinjection edema disappeared within three to four days of treatment.

In assessing clinical results, the investigators considered the degree of patient satisfaction (modest, fair, average, good, or excellent), the degree of observed clinical improvement, short- or long-term complications, and the possible need for implant removal. Improvement was deemed to be excellent by both physician and patient. No implant dislocation, implant migration, or other adverse reactions was noted.

To assess the biocompatability of BioAlcamid®, skin biopsy specimens were taken from human volunteers subjected to BioAlcamid® implants. Seven healthy male and female volunteers aged nineteen to thirty-seven years were evaluated. Each subject was injected with 0.5–1.0 cc of BioAlcamid® in the subcutaneous layer of the abdominal wall. Skin biopsy specimens were obtained three months after implantation. Light microscopic analysis of the skin specimens revealed fibroblasts located in the subcutaneous layer. These fibroblasts were arranged around a central amorphous core, representing the injected biomaterial, and were surrounded by a normal intercellular matrix showing no signs of inflammation. In the treated skin, the epidermis, dermis, and subcutaneous tissue adjacent to the filler were normal and identical to that of controls. Of great interest to the investigators were the observed connective fibrils that appeared to anchor the biomaterial to the deeper fibroblastic layer of the capsule that had formed at the capsule–implant interface. There were virtually no signs of neutrophil or monocyte tissue infiltration around the implant. The authors felt these confirmed that BioAlcamid® was a material highly compatible with human skin.

The authors further noted that BioAlcamid® was a permanent substance, without toxicity, was insoluble in tissue fluids, radiotransparent, and because of its high water content did not alter tissue consistency.

Although permanent in nature, they suggested the implant could be removed from human skin months to years after implantation.

In another study, eleven subjects with severe facial lipodystrophy secondary to HIV infection were evaluated. All, but one, were males; mean age was 48 (±7) years; mean HIV duration was 17 (±11) years. The subjects were randomly selected from patients seeking treatment for HLS. They came from different countries, including the United States, United Kingdom, Ireland, and Spain. All of the subjects had a full hematologic evaluation including full blood count, biochemistry, liver function, lipids, glucose, lactate, viral load, and CD4 cell count. All subjects had not received any prior treatment for their HLS. Patients who were receiving anticoagulant therapy, steroids, or diclofenac were not excluded from the study. Each of the subjects was injected bilaterally with 15–30 cc of BioAlcamid® into the subcutaneous regions of their buccal, malar, and temporal areas of the face. During the procedure, care was taken to inject the polymer superficially to the superficial musculoaponeurotic system (SMAS). Regional-injected anesthesia was used in conjunction with topical anesthesia in all treated subjects. The treated area was sculptured to obtain the best aesthetic appearance. Posttreatment antibiotics were given to all subjects. All of the subjects were first aesthetically assessed and then digitally photographed prior to injection after written informed consent had been obtained. The end point of treatment was achieved whenever the physician, nursing staff, and the subject all noted, and agreed, that the changes in facial contour had reached an optimal aesthetic outcome by visual observation. In addition to photographic documentation, all treated subjects had evaluation of their quality of life and psychological consequences of lipodystrophy investigated before and after treatment with a specifically designed social interaction questionnaire using a modified

Beck Depression Scale. Clinical improvement was evaluated three and eighteen months after treatment.

The subjects had a mean CD4 = 632/µl (±247), with a viral load below the limit of detection in 73 percent of the cases. All treated subjects noted that their quality of life improved dramatically three months after treatment. Four of the subjects felt that they had been able to obtain different employment as a direct result of undergoing the procedure. None of the subjects expressed regret at having undergone the procedure. All of the subjects showed a significant positive improvement in their social functioning ($P = 0.03$), and the modified Beck Depression Scale showed a mean overall score decrease from 14.57 to 10.21 after the procedure ($P = 0.1$). Almost all of the subjects reported that the results of the permanent filler became more natural in the weeks following the procedure. No treated subject reported any evidence of migration or nodules three months after treatment. The benefits of the biopolymer persisted at the eighteen-month evaluation.

MY TECHNIQUE

The ideal patient for BioAlcamid® treatment is one with significant facial lipoatrophy who seeks a permanent injectable treatment modality (Figure 12.1). Nevertheless, a variety of body sites have been injected (Table 12.1). BioAlcamid® is marketed as a frozen 4 percent acrylic alkylamide gel dissolved in 96 percent sterile water. It currently has CE clearance in Europe but has yet to receive FDA clearance in the United States.

Anesthesia is usually provided through localized nerve blocks. Currently used BioAlcamid® polyalkylamide gel, although injected into deep dermal and subcutaneous tissue, appears to be different from other dermal fillers, in that, once implanted, it becomes covered by a very thin collagen capsule (0.02 mm). This completely surrounds the gel,

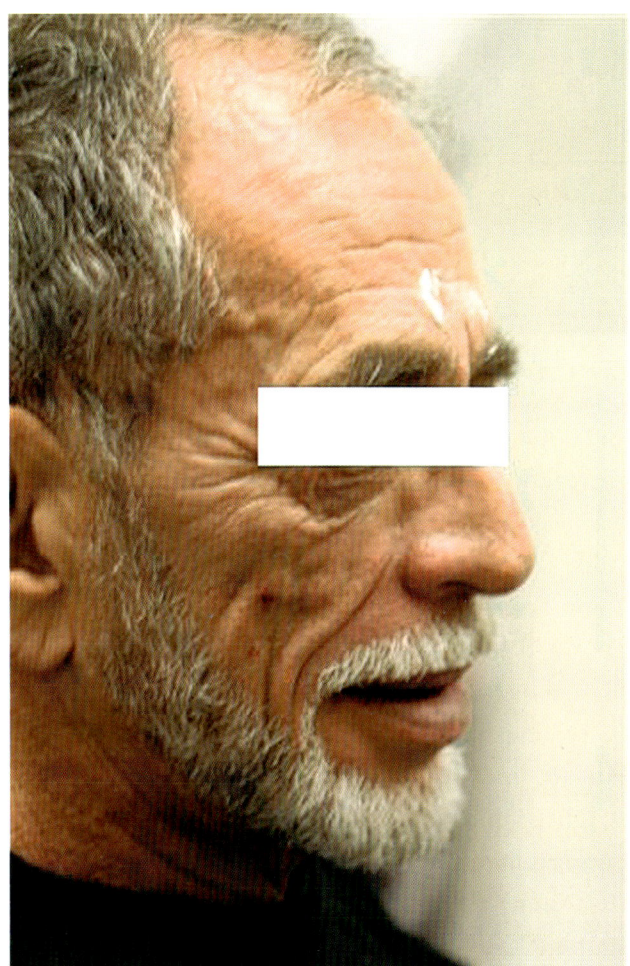

FIG. 12.1. *Ideal patient for BioAlcamid® injections.*

TABLE 12.1. BioAlcamid® Reported Injection Sites

Location	Authors
Face, legs, buttocks	Protopapa, C
Face	Treacy

isolating it from the host tissues and making it a type of endogenous prosthesis. According to Polymekon, the Italian manufacturer, the encapsulated prosthesis has the potential for later extraction from surrounding tissue. A variety of body sites can be injected with this permanent filler. To date, reactions to polyacrylamide gels appear to be rare and have not been reported in HLS-treated patients. The compound has been used since 2000 in over twenty countries

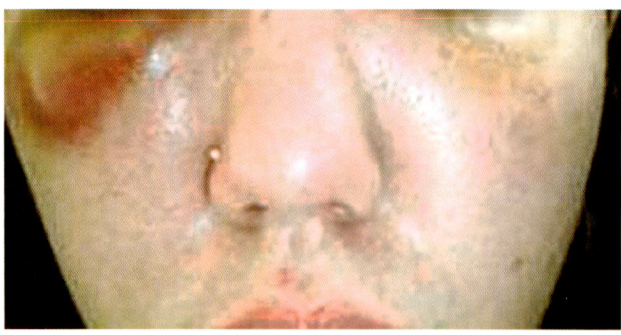

FIG. 12.2.   *Significant reaction to BioAlcamid® injections.*

and does not require any sensitization test as no allergic reaction has ever been reported. Although the gel has been extensively evaluated in a 2,000-patient study that demonstrated its safety, efficacy, and biocompatibility, there have been reports of occasional poorly defined adverse reactions. These reactions present as delayed hard nodular lesions that can only be removed with surgery. They can in fact be very difficult to remove (Figure 12.2).

Once implanted, BioAlcamid® forms a true permanent endoprosthesis, encompassed in a thin (0.02 mm), yet continuous fibrous capsule separating it from the host tissue. Although some have suggested that the prosthesis is easily removed, one must assume that with encapsulation, prosthesis removal may become increasingly more difficult.

What also has yet to be determined is whether this prosthesis is totally nonbiodegradable. Nonspecific free-radical processes are always functioning in the skin. Further safety studies will be required to determine whether there is specific enzymatic degradation of the prosthesis.

There also have now been reports of the potential for some permanent fillers to be associated with the onset of malignancies. Some have suggested that polyacrylamide permanent fillers, when injected into breast tissue, may induce breast carcinoma. It should be noted that such data are highly controversial. In addition, although polyacrylamide fillers are permanent in nature, they are quite different from the BioAlcamid® polyalkylamide filler. Nevertheless, such issues should raise caution about the use of any permanent filler in the breast.

REFERENCES

1. Protopapa, Sito, Caporale, Cammarota. BioAlcamid® in drug-induced lipodystrophy. *J Cosmet Laser Ther* 2003; **5**: 226–230.
2. Guaraldi G, Orlando G, De Fazio, D. Prospective, partially randomized, 24-week study to compare the efficacy and durability of different surgical techniques and interventions for the treatment of HIV-related facial lipoatrophy. 6th Lipodystrophy Workshop (6th IWADRLH), Washington. Abstract 12. *Antivir Ther* 2004; **9**: L9.
3. Formigli L, Zecchi S, Protopapa C, Caporale D, et al. BioAlcamid®: an electron electron microscopic study after skin implantation. *Plast Reconstr Surg* 2004; **113**: 1104–1106.
4. Pacini A, Ruggiero S, Morucci B, Cammarota SS, Protopapa B, Gulisano M. BioAlcamid®: a novelty for reconstructive and cosmetic surgery. *Ital J Anat Embryol* 2002; **107**: 209–214.
5. Pacini S, Ruggiero M, Cammrota N, Protopapa C, et al. BioAlcamid®, a novel prosthetic polymer, does not interfere with morphological and functional characteristics of human skin fibroblasts. *Plast Reconstr Surg* 2004; **113**: 1104–1106.
6. Treacy PJ, Goldberg DJ. Use of a biopolymer polyalkylamide filler for facial lipodystrophy in HIV-positive patients undergoing treatment with antiretroviral drugs. *Dermatol Surg* 2004; **32**: 804–808.

Chapter 13

COMBINATION OF APPROACHES IN AUGMENTATION FILLERS IN COSMETIC DERMATOLOGY

by

Susan H. Weinkle, MD and Harriet Lin Hall, ARNP

INTRODUCTION

Dermal filling agents and botulinum neurotoxin are currently widely utilized for facial augmentation and global restoration of the aging face. For years, the conventional wisdom regarding dermal injectables for facial rejuvenation was "Botox for the upper face; Fillers for the lower face." However, cosmetic dermatologists have advanced from the practice of treating single lines and wrinkles toward filling large facial areas to globally restoring natural facial contours (Ditre, 2008). Cosmetic dermatologists now have a better understanding of the facial aging process, and as new fillers become available, there is an increased recognition that when treating the aging face, the combination of soft tissue augmentation and botulinum toxin takes part in principal roles to fill, lift, tighten, and relax rhytids.

OVERVIEW OF INJECTABLE DERMAL FILLERS

Over the last four years, the US Food and Drug Administration (FDA) has approved many dermal filling agents. European countries and South America have had numerous dermal filling agents available for several years. Therefore, it can be quite difficult to decide what filler to use and where the filler should be injected. Injectable dermal fillers can be grouped according to their degree of degradability. In general, fillers may be classified into biodegradable and non-biodegradable products. The degradable material may be further classified into xenografts (derived from another species such as bovine collagen or hyaluronic acid of bacterial or avian origin), autografts (from the same person, such as autologous fat), and synthetic products (PLLA and CaHA) (Jones, 2007,

p. 106). Furthermore, combination products exist that include biodegradable as well as nonbiodegradable materials (polymethylmethacrylate, PMMA, suspended in bovine collagen). The following will be an overview of each group (Table 13.1).

BOVINE COLLAGEN

Before the introduction of the hyaluronic acids, collagen was the most widely used filler and was considered the gold standard with which other dermal fillers were compared. Injectable bovine collagen was FDA approved in 1981 as Zyderm collagen, which is 95 percent type I collagen and less than 5 percent type III collagen. Zyderm II was introduced in 1983 at a higher concentration of 65 mg/ml bovine collagen, and shortly following in 1985, Zyplast, which is cross-linked with glutaraldehyde to improve longevity, was launched. A disadvantage of bovine collagen is that 3 percent of individuals may display hypersensitivity. Double skin testing is now considered the standard of care.

Depending on the collagen content and the degree of cross-linking, different products should be used for different levels of the dermis. Zyderm I and Zyderm II (non–cross-linked) should be injected superficially into the papillary level of the dermis. Zyplast (cross-linked) should be injected more deeply into the reticular layer.

HUMAN COLLAGEN

Cosmoderm and Cosmoplast are natural human collagen grown in controlled laboratory conditions. These bioengineered collagen products were FDA approved in 2003 and do not require pretreatment testing. Cosmoderm, like Zyderm, consists of 35 mg/ml of collagen and is most useful for correcting fine lines. Cosmoplast, like Zyplast, consists of 65 mg/ml of collagen and is most useful for correcting mid-dermal defects such as nasolabial folds (Jones, 2007) (Figure 13.1A,B).

PORCINE COLLAGEN

The most recent addition to the injectable dermal collagen fillers is Evolence. Evolence was introduced in the European market in 2004 and recently FDA approved (June 2008) in the United States for treatment of nasolabial folds. In contrast to other collagens, this product is cross-linked by mimicking the process of collagen glycation using d-ribose as the cross-linking agent. One advantage over its counterparts is the removal of allergenic telopeptides, thus ensuring compatibility with human collagen; therefore, a skin testing is not required. Additionally, refrigeration is not required (Matarasso and Sadick, 2003) (Figure 13.2A,B).

TABLE 13.1. Biodegradable Fillers

Material	Origin	Products	
Collagen	Bovine	Zyderm, Zyplast	Allergan, Irvine, CA
	Porcine	Evolence	OrthoNeutrogena, Morris Plains, NJ
	Human (cultivated)	Cosmoderm, Cosmoplast	Allergan, Irvine, CA
	Human (self)	Autologen, Isologen	Isologen Inc., Houston, TX
Hyaluronic acid	Avian	Hylaform	Allergan, Irvine, CA
	Nonanimal	Restylane, Perlane, Juvaderm Ultra Prevelle Silk	Medicis, Scottsdale, AZ; Allergan, Irvine, CA; Mentor, Santa Barbara, CA
PLLA	Nonanimal	Sculptra	Dermik, Bridgewater, NJ
CaHA	Nonanimal	Radiesse	BioForm, San Mateo, CA
Fat	Human (self)	Fat	
Polyvinyl alcohol	Nonanimal	Bioinblue	

Note: Not all products available are listed. Not all products are FDA approved.

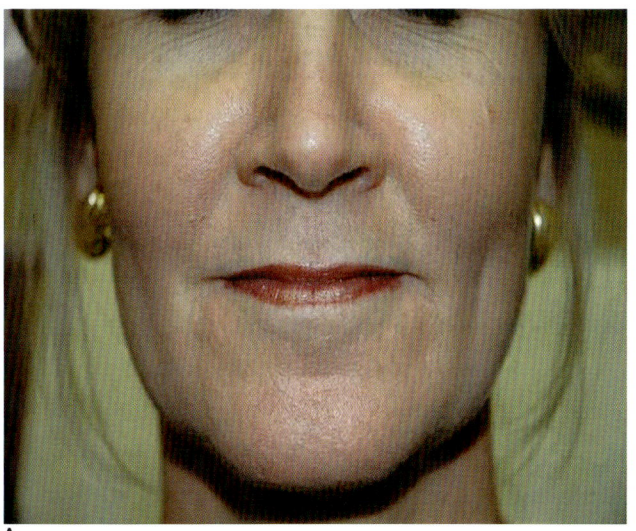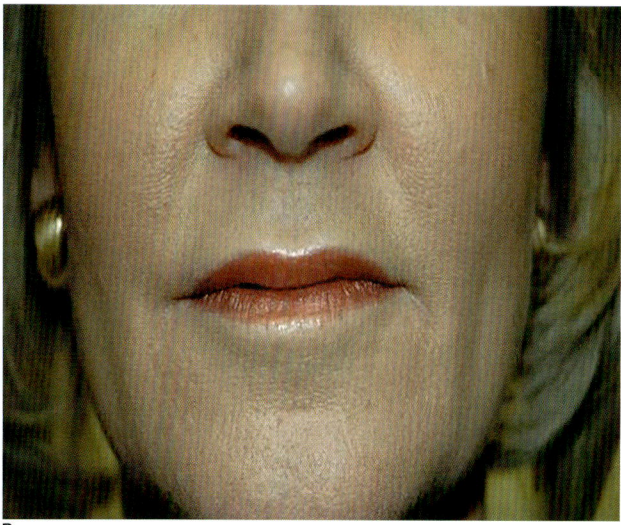

FIG. 13.1. *Lip augmentation with 1 cc of Cosmoderm in (A) vermilion borders and (B) body of the lip.*

HYALURONIC ACID

Hyaluronic acid fillers have rapidly become the new "gold" standard in soft tissue augmentation and are the fastest growing noninvasive aesthetic procedures in the United States according to the American Society for Aesthetic Plastic Surgery (Narins, Michaels, and Cohen, 2008, p. 31). Hyaluronic acid, which belongs to the family of glycosaminoglycans, consists of repeated disaccharide units and several variants are used as soft tissue fillers. Hyalans are ideal for patients who like the results of temporary tissue fillers but desire longer outcomes than collagen.

Hyaluronic acids can be derived from avian (dermis of nongender chicken combs) or bacterial fermentation (streptococcus bacteria). Several products with different viscosities and cross-linking have been adapted allowing the dermatologist a diverse range of injection depths.

The newest FDA-approved hyaluronic acid (Prevelle™ Silk) contains 0.3 percent of lidocaine to

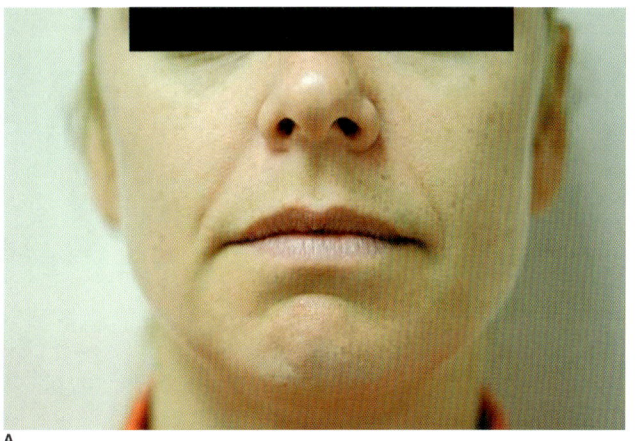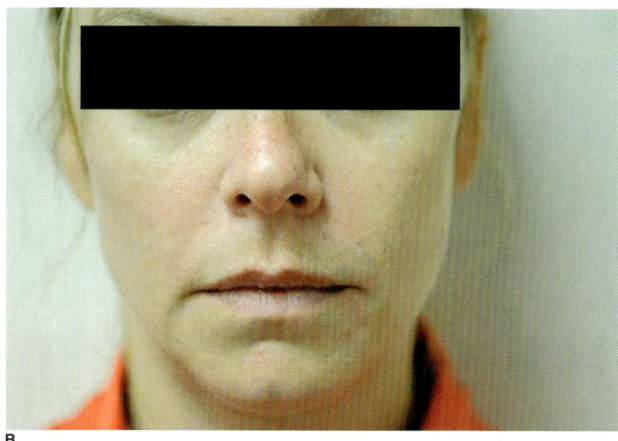

FIG. 13.2. *(A) Before nasolabial folds injected with Evolence 1.0 cc on each side. (B) Immediately after nasolabial folds injected with Evolence 1.0 cc on each side.*

minimize patient discomfort on injection however has less durability.

POLY-L-LACTIC ACID (PLLA)

Injectable PLLA is a biocompatible, resorbable polymer that results in an intended foreign body inflammatory response, dermal fibroplasia, and a slow metabolic degradation of the polymer microspheres as reported by Rotunda and Narins (2006, p. 151). Currently, PLLA is FDA approved only for HIV-mediated lipoatrophy. Double-blind studies for cosmetic use have been submitted to the FDA and are awaiting approval. When injected into the deep dermis, PLLA gradually stimulates collagen formation. The process can take time, and treatment sessions should be approximately four to six weeks apart. After reaching full correction, results can last up to two years.

Originally, the vial containing 150 mg PLLA freeze-dried powder was diluted with 3 ml sterile water at least two hours before injection. Current recommendations call for dilution with 5 ml or greater of diluent, and many authors recommend adding 1 ml of 2 percent lidocaine with epinephrine to decrease injection discomfort.

CALCIUM HYDROXYLAPATITE (CaHA)

Synthetic CaHA is a high-density, low-solubility bioceramic compound suspended in an aqueous gel carrier. After patient injected, the gel is absorbed and replaced with surrounding tissue structure forming a long-lasting implant composed of CaHA and natural tissue (Figure 13.3A,B). Unlike others fillers, CaHA does not require overcorrection, but since the matrix of a material acquires characteristics of the cells that populate after injection, precise placement is required for correction to occur. Skin testing is not necessary before use, and patients should be informed that the product may appear on facial X-ray (Carruthers and Carruthers, 2008, p. 87) (Figure 13.4).

POLYVINYL ALCOHOL

Polyvinyl alcohol is a comparatively newer biodegradable filler material. It consists of polyvinyl alcohol (8 percent) and water (92 percent). There have been no extensive clinical trials or larger case studies involving this product that have been published to date. Currently, polyvinyl alcohol has not been approved by the FDA (Table 13.2).

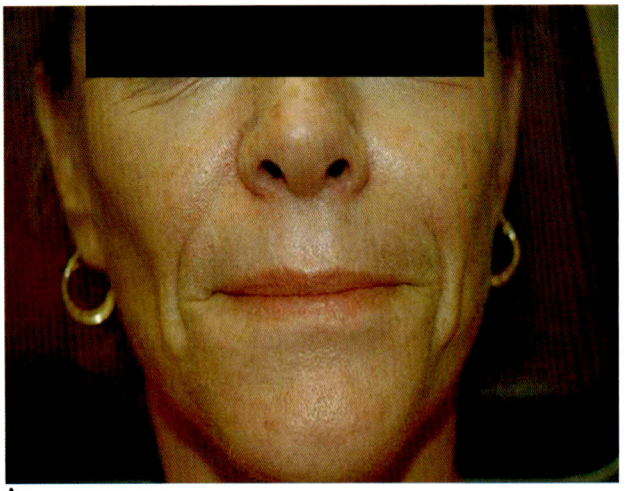
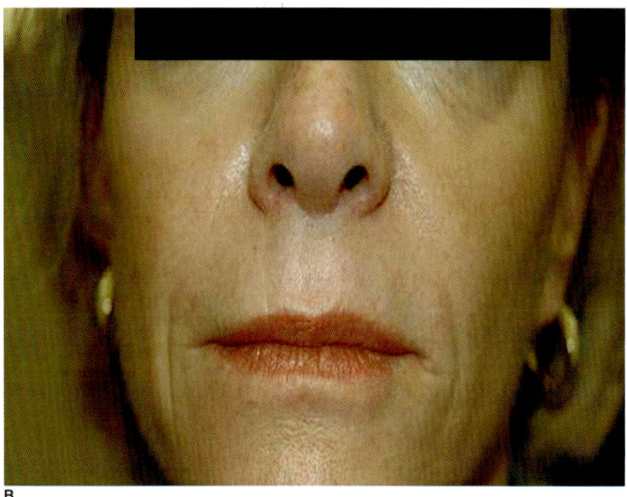

FIG.13.3.   (A) Before NLF correction with 2.6 cc CaHA. (B) After NLF correction with 2.6 cc CaHA.

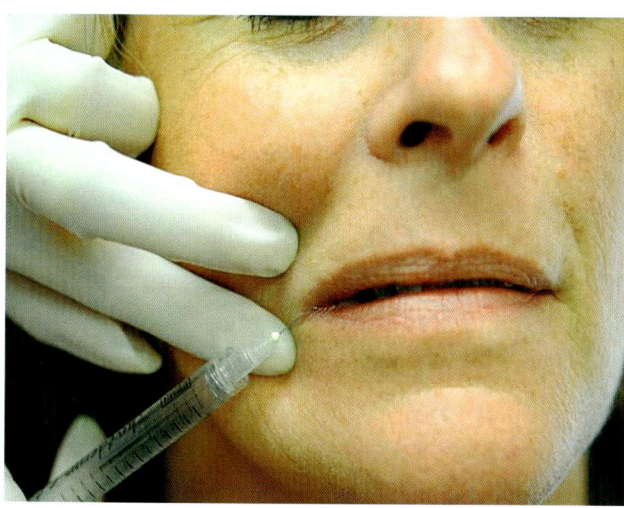

FIG. 13.4. *Preparing for injections at the corner of the lip and along the lower lateral corner of the lip.*

NONBIODEGRADABLE FILLERS

Several nonbiodegradable fillers are available, but none are approved by the FDA for cosmetic purposes. Nonbiodegradable fillers can be expensive and require excellent technique. To ensure patient satisfaction, patients should be thoroughly informed about the pros and cons of the suggested treatment.

Liquid injectable silicone (Silikon-1000, Adatosil 5000) was FDA approved in 1994 and 1997 as an injectable intraocular implant to treat retinal detachment.

Polyacrylamide (Aquamid®) is composed of 97.5 percent water and 2.5 percent cross-linked polyacrylamide. Bio-Alcamid™ is a permanent implant made from synthetic polyalkylimide. It should be injected into the subcutaneous layer. No prior skin testing is needed (Table 13.3).

TABLE 13.2. Nonbiodegradable Fillers

Material	Origin	Products	
Silicone	–	Silikon-1000	Alcon, Fort Worth, TX
Polyacrylamide	–	Aquamid	
Polyalkylimide	–	Bio-Alcamid	Polymekon, Italy

Note: No complete lists of products are available.

TABLE 13.3. Combination of Nonbiodegradable and Biodegradable Fillers

Temporary	Permanent	Products	
Collagen – bovine	PMMA	Artecoll/ ArteFill	Artes Medical Inc., CA
Hyaluronic acid	HEMA	Dermalive/ Dermadeep	

Note: Not all products available are listed.

PMMA

The combination of PMMA was introduced at the end of the 1980s; however, recent FDA approval (October 2008) of ArteFill® will make it the only permanent filler approved for use in the United States for cosmetic purposes. PMMA beads are suspended in a solution of 3.5 percent bovine collagen (delivery vehicle) and 0.3 percent lidocaine. Skin testing is required. ArteFill® is injected into the subdermis or at the deepest dermal level with a twenty-six- to twenty-seven-gauge needle using the tunneling technique. Targeted areas include deeper folds and rhytids. Overcorrection is not advisable and its permanence demands great care be taken in patient selection.

HYDROXYETHYL METHACRYLATE (HEMA) AND HYALURONIC ACID

HEMA and ethyl methacrylate microspheres suspended in hyaluronic acid have been available in Europe as Dermalive™ since the end of the 1990s. This product consists of 40 percent bacterial hyaluronic acid and 60 percent acrylic hydrogel particles. Dermalive™ should only be injected with a 27.5-gauge needle into the deeper layers of the dermis, at the junction between dermis and hypodermis, with a tunneling technique. Overcorrection should be avoided. It is also recommended that a period of at least three months should be left between two injection sessions (Rzany and Zielke, 2006, p. 7).

COMBINING SOFT TISSUE DERMAL FILLERS AND VOLUMIZERS

Soft tissue augmentation may be accomplished by surgery or by intradermal injections of biologic or synthetic implants. The latest developments in the realm of injectable fillers have made the greatest strides to eliminate granuloma formation, implant migration, short duration, and hypersensitivity reaction. As mentioned previously, there are a variety of filler formulations available for managing the aging phenomenon, and these may be used as monotherapy or multitherapy; offering patients only one or two filler options falls short of providing optimal management of the changes that accompany the aging face (Table 13.4). All individual fillers have their own unique profile in terms of approved uses, injection technique, durability, and adverse effects and may be more suitable for some applications than others (Monheit, 2008).

PATIENT EDUCATION

Preinjection Procedures

Before the injection of any filler, the patient should be counseled about what to expect in terms of any discomfort that may occur during or after injection, possible side effects, the results that he or she can expect, and the approximate durability of correction. Physicians who would like to successfully practice aesthetic medicine must understand that the vast majority of patients are unaware of what they really need. Pretreatment physician concerns include photographic documentation, patient's ability to understand the extent of correction possible, choosing the right product, and agreement on goals of treatment (e.g., cost, time frame, and return visits). Informed consent should be obtained. As with many dermatological procedures, patients should be advised to withhold any medication or supplement that might increase bleeding, for example, salicylate drugs, nonsteroidal anti-inflammatory drugs, high doses of vitamin E, and certain herbs (Jones, 2007).

Postinjection Procedures

Posttreatment photographs should be taken as soon as the injections have been completed and then taken again in ten to fourteen days. Postinjection placement of ice on the injection areas helps reduce and minimize tissue edema. Topical or oral administration of Arnica montana has natural anti-inflammatory effects that can sometimes help obviate bruising and swelling. Written post-op instructions are also helpful. For example, after a treatment of PLLA, massaging is

TABLE 13.4. Indications of Use – Soft Tissue Fillers

Filler	Type	Indications for Use
Cosmoderm®/Cosmoplast® (Inamed)	Purified collagen derived from human fibroblast cultures	Cosmoderm: fine line, wrinkles, shallow scars, also good for thin-skinned areas; cosmoPlast: deep lines, furrows, scars
Restylane®, Perlane® (Medicis)	Non–animal stabilized hyaluronic acid	Moderate-to-severe facial wrinkles and folds, that is, nasolabial folds
Juvederm Ultra® and Juvederm Ultra® Plus (Allergan)	Nonanimal hyaluronic acid	Moderate-to-severe facial wrinkles and folds, that is, nasolabial folds
Sculptra™ (Dermik Laboratories)	PLLA microparticles in suspension	Restoration and/or correction of the signs of facial fat loss
ArteFill® (Artes Medical)	PMMA microspheres suspended in bovine collagen gel	Correction of nasolabial folds
Radiesse® (BioForm)	CaHA microspheres in gel	Moderate-to-severe facial wrinkles and folds, including nasolabial folds; correction of facial fat loss
Evolence® (ColBar LifeScience)	Highly purified porcine collagen cross-linked via glymatrix	Moderate-to-severe facial wrinkles and folds

crucial. A postoperative "care card" dictating the massage regimen is helpful as well as the office phone number. Additionally, all cosmetic patients should have a follow-up phone call within two to three days of procedure to check on possible complications.

PROPER TECHNIQUE

Proper technique is paramount to optimize outcome and avoid complications with dermal filling agents. Infiltration of local anesthesia, needle size, injection technique, and multiple treatment sessions are important components to address before treating the patient. Other factors to consider when selecting a filler for a particular site include the durability of the filler, the level at which it is to be injected, and whether it is being used to add bulk or for layering. Accurate placement of the filler material is crucial (figure 159.1; Matarasso and Sadick, 2003, p. 2441). There are four injection techniques: serial multiple puncture, linear threading, fanning, and cross-hatching. The former deposits amounts of filler sequentially, with a small degree of overlap so that there are no spaces between the injected materials. Linear threading may use a retrograde technique where the full length of the needle is inserted into the proper dermal or subcutaneous plane and the filler is injected in a retrograde manner as the needle is withdrawn (Matarasso and Sadick, 2003, p. 2440). To fully appreciate the depth and scope of the facial defect, patients should be placed in a dependent or seated position with adequate lighting. Familiarity and experience are also important considerations for obtaining optimal results.

APPROACHES TO NONSURGICAL FACIAL REJUVENATION

The Structural Approach: Volumizing

PLLA, CaHA, and hyaluronic acid and botulinum toxin are easily combined for correction of the midface, nasolabial folds, jowl, chin, and lower cutaneous lip. As the dermatologist gains experience and the benefits of combining treatments including patient satisfaction become more apparent, combination therapy using different fillers naturally becomes a more familiar practice (Werschler, 2007, p. 12).

The following photographs illustrate how successful combining products can be. Numerous techniques aimed at restoring lost volume through the use of autologous and nonautologous fillers have demonstrated that rebalancing fat distribution or otherwise replacing volume to youthful proportions can restore the harmonious aesthetics of the face (Carruthers and Carruthers, 2005, p. 1605).

PLLA was used for global sculpting to initiate dermal thickening in the midface and bitemporal regions providing both a lifting and a filling effect. The injections are placed deep, preferably below the dermis. A fanning injection technique with cross-hatching is used to cover the midface to mid-to-upper facial regions. Because PLLA is commonly mixed with lidocaine at the time of injection, no other anesthetic agent is normally used other than topical anesthetic. PLLA requires a series of treatments. Therefore, complete volumizing is not attempted during the first session. Rather, a period of four to six weeks between treatments provides sufficient time for collagen formation and reevaluation for additional filling and sculpting of the treatment area. The duration of response to PLLA is the longest of dermal fillers/volumizers. PLLA may last approximately two years before needing a booster.

CaHA was used to correct the nasolabial folds and marionette lines. The correction achieved with CaHA is primarily the result of an immediate effect of the amount of material injected into the treatment area, although follow-up might be required. CaHA has a mild fibroblastic response that makes a comparatively minor contribution to the treatment response. By comparison, the response to PLLA is delayed and results from the fibroblastic response and collagen formation (Rendon, 2007, p. 8). Recently, the FDA approved porcine collagen (Evolence®). It is also a good choice for nasolabial folds filling and softening as it does not require a skin test and has less injection site reactions than HAs. Evolence is hydrophobic unlike the HAs, which are hydrophilic, and therefore results in less postinjection site edema. Complete correction can usually be achieved in a single visit, if desired. A finer version, Evolence™ Breeze, which has not yet been FDA approved, can be layered over Evolence in cases where there is a fine line overlying a deeper crease. Evolence™ Breeze is commonly used in lip augmentation (Smith, 2007, p. 391).

Hyaluronic acid was placed at the corners of the mouth (oral commissures), philtral columns, and upper/lower lip. The oral commissure is rebuilt at the level of the modiolus to provide a more youthful and relaxed appearance, with an uplifting that creates a hint of a smile. Placing injections along the philtral columns both enhances the cupid's bow area and redefines this important landmark of a youthful upper lip. The philtral columns are filled with recognition that they are not parallel in the vast majority of Caucasian patients. Rather, they form an inverted "V" shape that narrows as it approaches the columella of the nose (Werschler, 2008, p. 11).

With age, the lateral edges of the upper lip tend to hang over the lower lip at the point of the oral commissure. This creates a shadow and the appearance of a frown. To correct this, the skin is stiffened (Figure 13.4) at the corner of the mouth in preparation for injections at the corner of the lip and along the lower lateral corner of the lip. According to Klein (2005), adequate stretching of the lip is crucial because a firm surface improves the volume uniformity of flow of material, which can be hampered by the high viscosity of the agent.

The oblique folds extending from the lateral oral commissures to the edge of the mandible are called melomental folds or commonly referred to as marionette lines. The deeper they become, the more negative the resulting facial expression. These lines are formed by a loss of volume overlying the depressor anguli oris and platysma muscles. With the patient in a semisitting position, measure the depth of the fold by squeezing the lower cheek to the chin. This maneuver will give the clinician an estimate of volume of product needed. Mix CaHA with 2 percent lidocaine followed by introducing a twenty-eight-gauge needle, 3/4 inch at the lower angle of the triangular fold and injected with a retrograde tunneling type of linear threading technique, filling the triangles formed by the oral commissure and lower lip vermilion. These triangles are feathered with a serial puncture technique to produce volume correction of the groove and lip corners (Monheit and Prather, 2007, p. 403). It is important to keep the injection under and medial to the fold, as a lateral injection will actually increase the appearance of the fold. Additionally, the patient with significant elastosis benefits from injection at multiple layers to give adequate filling and prevent deep lumps. Posttreatment molding/massage should be performed to ensure the implant is evenly distributed, without nodules or irregularities.

TREATING FINE LINES AND LIP AUGMENTATION

Busso (2008) describes the periorbital region as the horseshoe-shaped area surrounding the eye and consists of the suborbital, zygoma, temporal, and brow areas. Although botulinum is used frequently to correct rhytids in the brow, combining fillers in this region can also aid in structural support, reduce excess skin, and improve the lateral lift of the brows. Aging of the periorbital region is characterized not only by the presence of rhytids (crow's feet) but also hollowing and skin laxity. Although botulinum toxin is often employed to correct rhytids in the brow, the use of fillers in this region can provide structural support, reduce excess skin, and improve lateral lift of the brows.

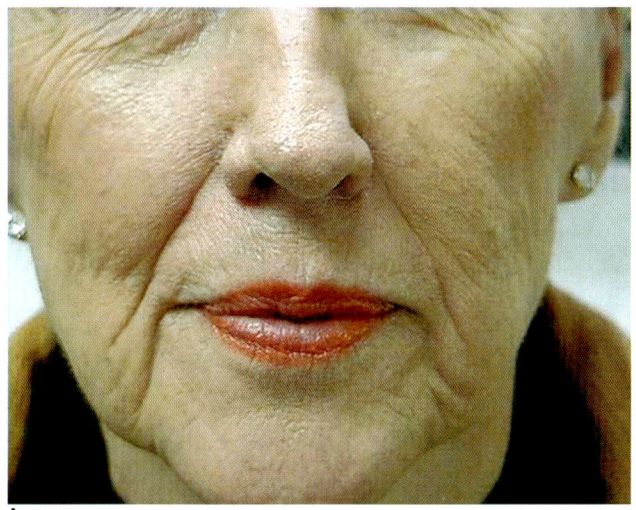 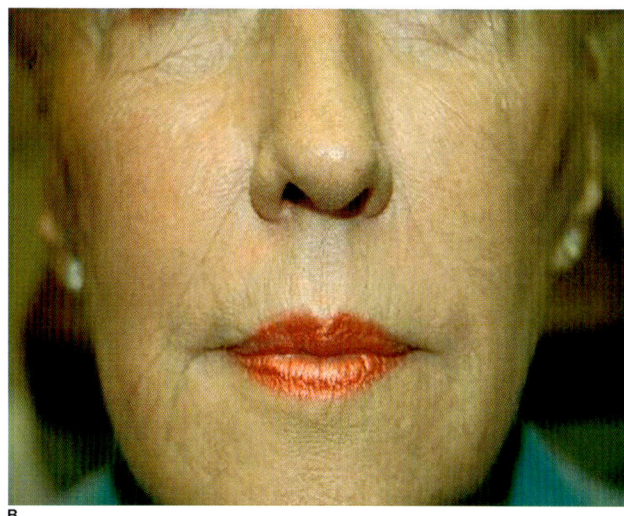

FIG. 13.5. *(A) Preinjection of zygoma region. (B) Postinjection of CaHA of zygoma region (3.6 cc).*

Because of the thinness of the skin and the proximity to the eyes, adroit use of fillers in the periorbital region requires greater skill and experience than in some other areas, for example, the nasolabial folds and marionette lines. The choice of filler is important. Many experienced dermatologic surgeons use PLLA in the temporal areas, HA-based products in the suborbital area, and CaHA in the area of the zygoma (Figure 13.5). Tear troughs can be treated with a combination of hyaluronic acid and collagen or PLLA, which promotes a longer lasting effect (Figure 13.6). This requires a deep injection given just above the periosteum. Bovine collagen may soon become a filler of the past due to its lack of durability and a single cross-linked HA can be used.

The lips are the center of the perioral frame. Although most patients initially request treatment for the lips alone, further education of the individual clarifies that if the perioral region is not treated, physicians will not be able to realize the full aesthetic potential of the entire lower face (Coleman and Carruthers, 2006, p. 177). It must be remembered that HA fillers are hygroscopic and may increase 10–15 percent in correction volume after injection unlike collagen, which loses volume. When injecting

the lips, the physician should note that upper versus lower lip volume is variable. As a general guideline, a ratio of lower to upper lip volume should be roughly 2:1. The lower lip is augmented by concentrating the injections along the central two-thirds of the central lip with the injections given into the core of the lip. The other variable when injecting lips with a hyaluronic acid is that hyaluronic acid is a stiffer product to inject compared to collagen. Additionally, the plunger pressure is slightly less. For smaller upper

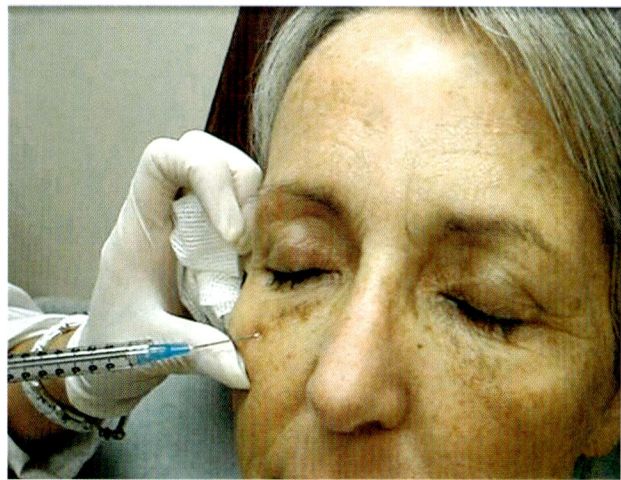

FIG. 13.6. *Injection of PLLA placed deeply into the tear trough region. Injection should not be given superficially to avoid "sausage roll appearance."*

lip rhytids, a direct injection of an HA into the rhytids will help soften the area. It is important to treat the complete perioral frame, vermilion lip, and the fine lines of the cutaneous lip. The key to the injection technique is to lay down a subdermal deposit of such double cross-linked HA so that the general contour is reestablished. A single cross-linked HA can then be subsequently layered for optimal sculpting (Carruthers and Carruthers, 2005, p. 1610).

TREATING ACNE SCARRING

Acne can produce many different types of skin defects, including inflammation and scarring. Scarring resulting from acne can be described as deep, shallow, wide, pitted, ice pick, depressed, hypotrophic, hypertrophic, or keloidal. The choice of technique for correction therefore is dependent on the type of scar or acne defect. Several techniques for facial acne scar revision have been described (Barnett and Barnett, 2005).

PLLA (Dermik Laboratories) is a long-acting volumizing device that restores volume and can reposition skin and tissue planes. PLLA acts to increase dermal thickness in a diffuse, stimulatory fashion; MOA is best suited to larger regions such as cheeks, temples, malar eminences rather than specific lines, wrinkles, or furrows. PLLA provides the foundation for treatment of atrophic acne scarring; then, layering with PMMA can commence.

ArteFill® (Artes Medical Inc., San Diego, CA) is the only permanent filler FDA approved for cosmetic use. It is a suspension of PMMA microspheres of 32–40 μm diameter in a 3.5 percent bovine collagen delivery vehicle, containing 0.3 percent lidocaine. After injecting the product, the collagen solution slowly dissolves leaving behind the nonbiodegradable PMMA microspheres that induce fibroplasias and become encapsulated by the patient's own collagen. Since ArteFill® is a permanent filler, overcorrection

may not be easily reversed. The patient should be educated that two to four sessions may be necessary before the final result is achieved. PMMA should be injected utilizing a linear threading technique into the deep dermis keeping the needle tip moving continuously and at the same time gently pressing on the plunger of the syringe. Patients hoping for immediate correction results that cannot be safely achieved within the first visit can have a layer of hyaluronic acid placed superior to the PMMA. As the hyaluronic acid slowly dissipates, additional PMMA injections will maintain a permanent correction.

According to Lemperle, (2003), Romano, and Busso PMMA is very effective for mature mildly depressed "rolling acne scars." These can be filled either horizontally from a distance of 5–10 mm or in "boxcar scars" perpendicularly downward directly into the center, continuously guiding the needle back and forth. In acne scars, PMMA should be implanted as superficially as possible until blanching appears. This effect can be spread and vanished with the fingernail. Recent acne scars should not be treated as the condition may become exacerbated. Ice pick scars require pretreatment. They should be punched, sutured, or subcised with a no. 11 blade or a double-beveled Nokor needle at a depth of approximately 1 mm. The fresh wound cavity can be easily filled with PMMA three to eight days later.

CONCLUSION

Many types of treatments are available for skin rejuvenation. Combining dermal fillers, volumizers, botulinum toxins, and light-based sources can expand treatment results and increase patient satisfaction. The science of soft tissue augmentation is evolving in an exponential manner. Keeping abreast of advances and perfecting a few techniques will be most advantageous for patients; it is not only what is injected but also how it is injected that determines the degree of success (Miller, Klein, and Lambros, 2001). It is an interesting period for the development of filling agents in the United States. The FDA has approved many new filling agents, others are still awaiting approval, and many others are undergoing clinical trials. Physicians across the country have begun using combinations of fillers to achieve the best results for our patients. It is important to remember that it is the dermatologist who will choose the right product, the right technique, and the right point in time for the patient.

REFERENCES

Barnett, J. and Barnett, C. (2005). Treatment of acne scars with liquid silicone injections: 30 year perspective. *Dermatologic Surgery,* **21**, 1542–1549.

Busso, M. (2008). Soft tissue augmentation: nonsurgical approaches to treatment of the mid and lower facial regions. *Dermatology Nursing,* **20**, 211–219.

Carruthers, J. and Carruthers, A. (2008). Fillers Working By Fibroplasias: Radiesse. In: Carruthers, J., Carruthers, A. (Eds.) *Soft Tissue Augmentation.* Saunders, Philadelphia, pp. 87–89.

Carruthers, J.D. and Carruthers, A. (2005). Facial sculpting and tissue augmentation. *Dermatologic Surgery,* **31**, 1604–1612.

Coleman, K.R. and Carruthers, J. (2006). Combination therapy with Botox and fillers: the new rejuvenation paradigm. *Dermatologic Therapy,* **19**, 177–188.

Ditre, C.M. (2008). Dermal fillers for facial rejuvenation and restoration: integrating new therapies into clinical practice. *Cosmetic Dermatology,* **21**(Suppl. 2 S1), 11–14.

Jones, D. (2007). Dermal Fillers. In: Goldberg, D. (Ed.) *Facial Rejuvenation.* Springer, New York, pp. 106–123.

Klein, A.W. (2005). In search of the perfect lip: 2005. *Dermatologic Surgery,* **31**, 1599–1603.

Lemperle, G., Romano, J., and Busso, M. (2003). Soft tissue augmentation with Artecoll: 10 year history, indications, techniques, and complications. *Dermatologic Surgery,* **29**, 573–587.

Matarasso, S.L. and Sadick, N.S. (2003). Soft tissue augmentation. In: *Dermatology.* Mosby, New York City, pp. 2439–2449.

Miller, T., Klein, A., and Lambros, V. (2001). Soft tissue augmentation. *Journal of Aesthetic Surgery,* **20**, 309–314.

Monheit, G. and Prather, C. (2007). Hyaluronic acid fillers for the male patient. *Dermatologic Therapy,* **20**, 394–406.

Monheit, G.D. (2008). Dermal fillers for facial rejuvenation and restoration: integrating new therapies into clinical practice. *Cosmetic Dermatology,* **21**(Suppl. 2 S1), 7–10.

Narins, R., Michaels, J., and Cohen, J. (2008). Hylans and Soft Tissue Augmentation. In: Carruthers, J., Carruthers, A. (Eds.) *Soft Tissue Augmentation.* Saunders Elsevier, Philadelphia, pp. 31–50.

Rendon, M. (2007). Nonsurgical total facial restoration: combining therapies for optimal patient outcomes: a case study approach. *Cosmetic Dermatology,* **20**(Suppl. 2 S1), 6–8.

Rotunda, A. and Narins, R. (2006). Poly-L-lactic acid: a new dimension in soft tissue augmentation. *Dermatologic Therapy,* **19**, 151–158.

Rzany, B. and Zielke, H. (2006). Overview of Injectable Fillers. In: de Maio, M., Rzany, B. (Eds.) *Injectable Fillers in Aesthetic Medicine*: Springer, Berlin, pp. 1–9.

Smith, K. (2007). New fillers for the new man. *Dermatologic Therapy,* **20**, 388–393.

Werschler, W.P. (2008). Dermal fillers for facial rejuvenation and restoration: integrating new therapies into clinical practice. *Cosmetic Dermatology,* **21**(Suppl. 2 S1), 3–7.

Werschler, W.P. (2007). Nonsurgical total facial restoration: combining therapies for optimal patient outcomes: a case study approach. *Cosmetic Dermatology,* **20**(Suppl. 2 S1), 9–13.

Chapter 14

FILLING COMPLICATIONS

by

Papri Sarkar, MD and Ranella J. Hirsch, MD

INTRODUCTION

Slowing down the inevitable course of skin aging has been a popular notion for hundreds of years. Ancient Egyptians compounded early chemical peels using the lactic acid in milk and performed an early form of microdermabrasion with salt, alabaster, and animal oils.[1] More sophisticated methods including soft tissue augmentation with autologous fat were first reported in the German literature by Neuber in 1893.[2]

The first U.S. Food and Drug Administration (FDA)–approved filler was bovine collagen (Zyderm I) in 1981. Since then, a myriad of soft tissue fillers have been introduced. These include both bovine and human collagens (Zyderm, Zyplast, CosmoDerm, and CosmoPlast), hyaluronic acids (Restylane, Perlane, Juvederm, and Hylaform), calcium hydroxyapatite (Radiesse), poly-l-lactic acid (Sculptra), and synthetic polymers such as liquid silicone and Artecoll or Artefill. These procedures have gained popularity as they are generally safe in experienced hands, and many show rapid improvement yielding high levels of clinical satisfaction.[3]

All cosmetic procedures have associated risks. As the incidence of soft tissue augmentation has increased, as would be expected, adverse effects have been reported more commonly. In a survey of 286 patients, McCraken et al. recently reported a 5 percent complication rate among ophthalmologists performing soft tissue augmentation procedures.[4] This article will emphasize the prevention, identification, and treatment complications with a focus on temporary fillers. Permanent fillers (such as Artecoll) permit greater longevity with which comes the greater risk of adverse sequelae. These permanent substances present a greater risk of causing late-onset (>one year) granulomas.

PREOPERATIVE

A critical step of any cosmetic procedure takes place before the dermatologist ever touches the patient. Patients must be carefully screened, consented, and given realistic expectations as to results and potential complications. If a "preview" of the corrected effect is desired, a small volume of lidocaine or normal saline may be injected to simulate volume replacement.[5] This is of particular value with the first-time dermal filler patient.

After determining that a patient is indeed a good candidate for soft tissue augmentation, great care should be taken to assess and document facial asymmetry. Lesions that might be made more prominent posttreatment should be identified. These characteristics should be pointed out to the patient and standardized pre- and postprocedure photographs taken. Patients should be asked about a history of cold sores as herpes simplex virus (HSV) infection can be reactivated and carries the risk of dyspigmentation and/or scarring. Standard practice is to prescribe prophylactic antivirals several days preprocedure for patients at risk.

COMPLICATIONS

Ecchymoses, Tenderness, and Edema

Erythema, swelling, and ecchymoses are common and predictable side effects with the injection of dermal fillers. Any or all can occur during, immediately following, or hours after the injections are administered. Edema following the use of collagen-based products is more immediate than the edema after the use of the hydrophilic hyaluronans. Given the rich vascular supply of the face, it is not surprising that patients may also experience bruising after injection. This is typically minor and resolves without intervention after two to three days.

More significant ecchymoses may develop in patients who drink alcohol and take blood thinners (including coumadin and nonsteroidal anti-inflammatory drugs) or certain herbal medications associated with prolonged bleeding. Examples include vitamin E, feverfew, ginger, garlic, ginseng, and gingko. The prevalent use of such supplements necessitates diligent pretreatment questioning as they are often underreported by patients who do not associate them with untoward effects. Ciocon et al. recommend discontinuing these agents at least one week before a major surgery, although

bleeding time may take two to three weeks to correct fully.[6] Gladstone and Cohen have reported that the fanning injection technique for dermal fillers can also increase the likelihood of intraprocedural bleeding as well.[7]

Another herbal preparation, arnica, is extracted from Arnica montana of the Asteraceae family[8] and is anecdotally reported to decrease bleeding and swelling. However, two recent randomly controlled trials did not find evidence of this. In the first, Seeley et al. used a computer software program to grade ecchymoses in patients pretreated with arnica or placebo for face-lifts. Although those patients pretreated with arnica were graded as having less ecchymoses by the computer program, both the patients and the physicians in this group did not appreciate a clinical difference.[8]

In the second reference, Totonchi's group found that although arnica improved postoperative edema, it was not effective in reducing ecchymoses postrhinoplasty.[9]

Cross-linked collagen-related peptide has been shown to induce platelet aggregation and stabilization.[10] This finding, along with the collected clinical experience of many cosmetic dermatologists, supports the notion that the collagen-based fillers may be associated with decreased bruising.[11] However, this finding has not been formally investigated.

LOCATION, LOCATION, AND LOCATION

Of key importance with all filler materials is making sure that one introduces it in its proper target space. Generally, human collagen should be injected into the mid-dermis. The target for medium-length hyaluronic acid fillers such as Restylane and Juvederm is the deep dermis.[12] Calcium hydroxyapatite (Radiesse) should be injected at the dermal–subcutaneous border.[13,14] Fat and poly-l-lactic acid should be placed deeper in the subcutis.[15]

HIGH-RISK SITES, NECROSIS, AND SUPERFICIAL BEADING

It is crucial for the injecting physician to have a detailed knowledge of the relevant anatomy. The small-caliber arteries of common facial injection sites have little collateral circulation and are thus at increased risk for occlusion. The glabella is the highest risk area and has been the most common site reported to be associated with necrosis with any filler.[16,17]

Zyderm I is a bovine collagen filler formulated at 35 mg/ml but in contrast to Zyplast can be used in the glabellar area. Zyplast is cross-linked by the addition of glutaraldehyde to make it more resistant to degradation. Increasing the size of the particles by cross-linkage leads to a higher likelihood of vascular occlusion especially of the thin-caliber vessels of the glabella.[18] Zyderm II, also a bovine collagen formulated at 65 mg/ml, was reported to cause amaurosis following injection into the glabella. This was believed to be due to occlusion of the retinal artery.[19]

Tissue necrosis, a rare but clinically important potential complication, has occurred most commonly following soft tissue augmentation of the glabella. This may be due to occlusion of minute vessels branching from the relatively superficial supratrochlear and supraorbital arteries that provide the blood supply to the glabella, a region with limited collateral blood flow. Tissue viability may be compromised when arterial circulation is impaired by intravascular thrombosis or extravascular compression exerted by a mass of filler material upon these watershed vessels.[20] Schanz et al. reported a case of necrosis after glabellar injection of Restylane.[21]

Should vascular compromise be suspected, as evidenced by a significant area of blanching, ecchymosis, or reticulated erythema during or after injection, a recent protocol[20] suggests immediate discontinuance of injections and the encouragement of quick

vasodilatation by gentle massage, the immediate application of heat (hot water on gauze), and tapping the distribution of the vessels to facilitate flow. The application of nitroglycerin paste (optimally under occlusion) can also produce vasodilatation.

Off-label use of hyaluronidase, a product approved by the FDA, offers another useful therapeutic strategy. Brody reported on formulations of hyaluronidase that can be obtained including compounded product as well as Vitrase and Amphadase.[22] Hyaluronidase is a soluble protein enzyme that hydrolyzes hyaluronic acid by splitting the glucosaminidic bond between C1 of the glucosamine moiety and C4 of glucuronic acid. Adverse reactions to hyaluronidase are uncommon and when reported are most frequently local injection site reactions. If signs of impending injection necrosis following injection of a hyaluronic acid–type filler (i.e., Restylane [Medicis Aesthetics, Inc., Scottsdale, AZ, USA], Hylaform or Hylaform Plus [INAMED Aesthetics, Santa Barbara, CA, USA], Captique [INAMED Aesthetics], Juvederm [INAMED Aesthetics]) occur, hyaluronidase can be used to diffuse the hyaluronic acid gel–injected material.[23,24]

Any filler that is not injected at the appropriate depth may lead to beading or clumping. Agents such as hyaluronic acid or calcium hydroxyapatite may cause a blue–white color if injected too superficially. This is known as the Tyndall or Rayleigh effect.[25] The Tyndall effect is due to light scattering. The "color" of an object is determined by how much light of a certain wavelength is being reflected to us or scattered for our eyes to see. Light with shorter wavelengths, such as blue, scatters more readily than that with longer wavelengths. The longer wavelength red light, which penetrates deeper into the skin, gets absorbed by substances in the skin, such as blood. Once absorbed, there is less red light available to scatter. If a filler is injected too superficially, the red light penetrates through it, while the blue light is reflected to our eyes as scatter so the substance appears blue.[26,27]

The incidence of this side effect is most likely to occur if using a filler meant to be injected deep into the skin (e.g., calcium hydroxyapatite) within an area of limited dermis or subcutaneous tissue. These high-risk areas include the so-called "I" zone of the central face: the nasojugal folds, nasal dorsum, and lip. Periorbital and perioral rhytids or "crow's feet" and "pucker lines" should also be included in this group as substances need to be injected relatively superficially in these areas. Other sites of concern are forehead rhytids, which may be associated with ridging on either side and even the nasolabial folds.

Hirsch recently published a report on correcting superficially placed hyaluronic acid (Juvederm) in the nasojugal fold. Management options include tincture of time, needle incision with an 11 blade to express the product, laser therapy with a 1,064-nm Q-switched Nd:YAG,[28] or the use of hyaluronidase. Hyaluronidase, a non–ATP requiring enzyme that dissolves hyaluronic acid in the skin, has proven to be an invaluable agent in the management of excessive hyaluronic acid placement.[29]

ALLERGIC REACTIONS/ HYPERSENSITIVITY

One disadvantage of bovine-derived collagen products is their potential for immunogenicity; thus, before injection with either Zyderm or Zyplast, documentation of two negative skin tests is recommended before initiating treatment with these products.[30] Overall, the incidence of allergy to bovine collagens has been estimated at 1–5 percent.[30] Signs of hypersensitivity include erythema, edema, induration, pain, and/or pruritus. Double skin allergy testing performed two weeks apart is recommended for bovine collagen products. It may be performed with commercially available Zyderm test syringes. Allergy to

lidocaine or bovine collagen is a contraindication to testing or treatment.[31]

Friedman et al. reviewed the safety data for the non–animal stabilized hyaluronic acid fillers Restylane, Perlane, and Restylane Fine Lines, products made via bacterial fermentation process. The authors note that in 1999, hypersensitivity was the major reaction in 1 in every 1,400 patients. This was believed to be secondary to impurities introduced during the bacterial fermentation process. In 2000, this number dropped to 1 in 5,000 and was believed to be due to the introduction of a more purified hyaluronic acid raw material. The average time of onset and duration were twenty-two and fifteen days, respectively.

The authors noted that in general, the reactions self-resolved in one to two days on the face and after one week in the lips. Antecedent skin testing is not performed for these agents and rates of hypersensitivity have decreased rapidly as purification techniques have improved.[32] Hyaluronidase injections help speed up the resolution of these hypersensitivity reactions by breaking down the product more rapidly[11] but hypersensitivity to this agent must be kept in mind as well. Hyaluronidase may elicit an immediate or delayed hypersensitivity reaction, and in very rare cases, angioedema has been reported.[33–35]

GRANULOMAS

Granulomas may occur in 0.01–0.1 percent of the patient population and are most common in patients injected with nonbiodegradable or slowly biodegradable fillers.[36] They generally appear within six months of injection but may occur as late as twenty-four months postinjection.[37,38] In general, they are treated with steroids. Lemperle et al. recommend intralesional steroids and note that the initial dose must be high despite a 20–30 percent rate of skin atrophy. The authors write that "starting with low doses of triamcinolone (5–10 mg/ml) seems to create resistance and increases the risk of recurrence." They suggest blanching injections of a 40 mg/ml ampule of kenalog followed by the same or double dose if disappearance of the granuloma is not noted after three to four weeks. Other treatments they suggest include 1) intralesional betamethasone 5–7 mg or 2) undiluted methyl-prednisolone 20–40 mg or 3) 1/3 diprosone (1.1 mg) + 1/3 5-fluorouracil (1.6 ml) + 1/3 lidocaine (1 ml) or 4) kenalog (10 mg/ml) + 5-fluorouracil (50 mg/ml). Minocycline has been reported to be beneficial in the treatment of silicone granulomas[39] and a combination of intralesional steroids and 5-fluorouracil has also been tried.[40] Lemperle et al. suggest surgical excision as a last resort generally reserved for granulomas on the lips or those in the subcutaneous fat.[38]

INFECTION

Infection is a rare and early complication after injection with fillers. Tender, warm, erythematous fluctuant nodules may appear along the injection site. The patient may have systemic symptoms such as fever or chills. Usually, *Staphylococcus aureus* is the causative organism, although sterile abscesses and mycobacteria have also been reported.[7] As mentioned previously, reactivation of HSV may also occur and the standard of care is to treat patients with a history of HSV with preoperative antivirals.

MIGRATION AND MISPLACEMENT

Migration has been reported with nonbiodegradable fillers such as Artecoll or liquid silicone. Repositioning or removal of implant is the recommended treatment.[3] Migration has not yet been described with the temporary fillers.

Misplacement of the biodegradable fillers may be contoured with manual manipulation with the wooden end of a cotton-tipped applicator as described by Duffy.[5] With the hyaluronans, the judicious use of hyaluronidase may help as well. Injection of too much hyaluronidase in one area may cause a cycle of asymmetry or overcorrection and undercorrection. For this reason, before injection, we recommend discussing this possible side effect frankly, especially with patients who desire a very "full" appearance to lips or folds. After injection, if the patient still prefers more volume, more product can be injected into the area, but patients must be made aware beforehand if additional fees apply.

CONCLUSION

In soft tissue augmentation and medicine in general, prevention is still the best medicine. Before augmentation, the injector should be well versed in product options and limitations, appropriately trained in injection techniques, and have a strong awareness of the relevant anatomic landmarks. Frank review of applicable risks before injection is mandatory. When complications occur, the patient should be seen as soon as possible, and open discussion regarding possible treatment options as outlined above should take place. We find that open dialogue with patients in combination with prudent use of fillers leads to satisfied patients and physicians.

REFERENCES

1. Monheit GD, Chastain MA. Chemical and mechanical skin resurfacing. In: Bolognia JL, Jorizzo JL, Rapini RP, eds. *Dermatology*, 1st edn. Elsevier Saunders: Philadelphia, 2003; 2379–2381.

2. Klein AW. Techniques for soft tissue augmentation: an "a to z". *Am J Clin Dermatol* 2006; 7(2):107–120.

3. De Bouelle K. Management of complications after implantation of fillers. *J Cosmet Dermatol* 2004; 3(1):2–15.

4. McCraken MS, Khan JA, Wulc AE, et al. Hyaluronic acid gel (Restylane) filler for facial rhytides: lessons learned from American Society of Ophthalmic Plastic and Reconstructive Surgery member treatment of

286 patients. *Ophthal Plast Reconstr Surg* 2006; **22**: 188–191.

5. Duffy DM. Complications of fillers: overview. *Dermatol Surg* 2005; **31**:1626–1633.

6. Ciocon JO, Ciocon DG, Galindo DJ. Dietary supplements in primary care. *Geriatrics* 2004; **59**(9): 20–24.

7. Gladstone HB, Cohen JL. Adverse effects when injecting facial fillers. *Semin Cutan Med Surg* 2007; **6**:34–39.

8. Seeley BM, Denton AB, Ahn MS, Maas CS. Effect of homeopathic Arnica montana on bruising in face-lifts. *Arch Facial Plast Surg* 2006; **8**:54S–59S.

9. Totonchi A, Guyuron B. A randomized, controlled comparison between Arnica and steroids in the management of postrhinoplasty ecchymosis and edema. *Plast Reconstr Surg* 2007; **120**:271–274.

10. Smethurst PA, Onley DJ, Jarvis GE, et al. Structural basis for the platelet-collagen interaction: the smallest motif within collagen that recognizes and activates platelet glycoprotein VI contains two glycine–proline–hydroxyproline triplets. *J Biol Chem* 2007; **282**(2): 1296–1304.

11. Baumann L. Dermal fillers. *J Cosmet Dermatol* 2004; **3**:249–250.

12. Narins RS, Brandt F, Leyden J, et al. A randomized, double-blind multicenter comparison of the efficacy and tolerability of Restylane versus Zyplast for the correction of nasolabial folds. *Dermatol Surg* 2003; **29**:588–595.

13. Berlin A, Cohen JL, Goldberg DJ. Calcium hydroxyapatite for facial rejuvenation. *Semin Cutan Med Surg* 2006; **25**:132–137.

14. Roy D, Sadick N, Mangat D. Clinical trial of a novel filler material for soft tissue augmentation of the face containing synthetic calcium hydroxyapatite microspheres. *Dermatol Surg* 2006; **32**:1134–1139.

15. Vleggaar D. Soft tissue augmentation and the role of poly-L-lactic acid. *Plast Reconstr Surg* 2006; **118**: 46S–54S.

16. Hanke CW, Higley HR, Jolivette DM, Swanson NA, Stegman SJ. Abscess formation and local necrosis after treatment with Zyderm or Zyplast collagen implant. *J Am Acad Dermatol* 1991; **25**:319–326.

17. Schanz S, Schippert W, Ulmer A, Rassner G, Fierlbeck G. Arterial embolization caused by injection of hyaluronic acid (Restylane). *Br J Dermatol* 2002; **146**:928–929.

18. Baumann LS, Daza I, Lourenco AC, Lazarus M. Cosmetic dermatology. In Marks R, Leyden JL, eds. *Dermatologic Therapy in Current Practice,* 1st edn. Elsevier Saunders: Philadelphia, 2001; 237.

19. Castillo GD. Management of blindness in the practice of cosmetic surgery. *Otolaryngol Head Neck Surg* 1989 Jun **100**(6):559–562.

20. Glaich AS, Cohen JL, Goldberg LH. Injection necrosis of the glabella: protocol for prevention and treatment after use of dermal fillers. *Dermatol Surg* 2006; **32**(2):285–290.

21. Schanz S, Schippert W, Ulmer A, et al. Arterial embolization caused by injection of hyaluronic acid (Restylane®). *Br J Dermatol* 2002; **146**:928–929.

22. Brody HJ. Use of hyaluronidase in the treatment of granulomatous hyaluronic acid reactions or unwanted hyaluronic acid misplacement. *Dermatol Surg* 2005; **31**(8):893–897.

23. Hirsch RJ, Lupo M, Cohen JL, Duffy D. Delayed presentation of impending necrosis following soft tissue augmentation with hyaluronic acid and successful management with hyaluronidase. *J Drugs Dermatol* 2007; **6**(3):325–328.

24. Hirsch RJ, Cohen JL, Carruthers JD. Successful management of an unusual presentation of impending necrosis following a hyaluronic acid injection embolus and a proposed algorithm for management with hyaluronidase. *Dermatol Surg* 2007; **33**(3):357–360.

25. Hirsch RJ, Narurkar V, Carruthers J. Management of injected hyaluronic acid induced Tyndall effects. *Lasers Surg Med* 2006; **38**:202–204.

26. Suhai B, Horvath G. How well does the Rayleigh model describe the E-vector distribution of skylight in clear and cloudy conditions? A full-sky polarimetric study. *J Opt Soc Am A Opt Image Sci Vis* 2004; **21**(9): 1669–1676.

27. Anderson RR. Rest azured? *J Am Acad Dermatol* 2001; **44**(5):874–875.

28. Hirsch RJ, Narurkar V, Carruthers JD. Management of hyaluronic acid induced Tyndall effects. *Lasers Surg Med* 2006; **38**(3):202–204.

29. Hirsch RJ, Brody HJ, Carruthers JD. Hyaluronidase in the office: a necessity for every dermasurgeon that injects hyaluronic acid. *J Cosmet Laser Ther* 2007; **9**(3):182–185.

30. Klein AW. Skin filling. Collagen and other injectables of the skin. *Dermatol Clin* 2001; **19**:491–508.

31. Matarrasso SL. The use of injectable collagens for aesthetic rejuvenation. *Semin Cutan Med Surg* 2006; **25**(3):151–157.

32. Friedman PM, Mafong EA, Kauvar ANB, Geronemus RG. Safety data of injectable nonanimal stabilized hyaluronic acid gel for soft tissue augmentation. *Dermatol Surg* 2002; **28**:491–494.

33. Eberhart AH, Weiler CR, Erie JC. Angioedema related to the use of hyaluronidase in cataract surgery. *Am J Ophthalmol* 2004; **138**:142–143.

34. Agrawal A, McLure HA, Dabbs TR. Allergic reaction to hyaluronidase after a peribulbar injection. *Anesthesia* 2003; **58**:493–494.

35. Ahluwalia HS, Lukaris A, Lane CM. Delayed allergic reaction to hyaluronidase: a rare sequel to cataract surgery. *Eye* 2003; **17**(2):263–266.

36. Nicolau PJ. Long-lasting and permanent fillers: biomaterial influence over host tissue response. *Plast Reconstr Surg* 2007; **119**:2271–2286.

37. Alcalay J, Alkalay R, Gat A, Yorav S. Late-onset granulomatous reaction to Artecoll. *Dermatol Surg* 2003; **29**(8):859–862.

38. Lemperle G, Rullan PP, Gauthier-Hazan N. Avoiding and treating dermal filler complications. *Plast Reconstr Surg* 2006; **118**:92S–107S.

39. Senet P, Bachelez H, Ollivaud L, Vignon-Pennamen D, Dubertret L. Minocycline for the treatment of cutaneous silicone granulomas. *Br J Dermatol* 1999; **140**(5):985–987.

40. Blugerman G, Schacelzon D, Dreszman R. Intralesional use of 5-FU in subcutaneous fibrosis. *J Drugs Dermatol* 2003; **2**:169–171.

Chapter 15

POSTPROCEDURE MANAGEMENT AND PATIENT INSTRUCTIONS

by

Andrew A. Nelson, MD and Joel L. Cohen, MD

INTRODUCTION

With the unprecedented rise in the use of inject-able fillers, an increasing number of patients are approaching their physicians to undergo soft tissue augmentation. It is absolutely essential to educate patients about the procedure, its potential bene-fits, and its potential complications. As always, this should be done prior to the procedure to be most effective. Detailed pre- and postprocedure instruc-tions are an essential part of this education process. It is this education that ultimately empowers pati-ents and helps them to achieve their ideal cosmetic outcome.

Effectively written pre- and postprocedure instruc-tions serve multiple important functions in educating patients regarding their cosmetic procedures. First and foremost, the instructions help patients to under-stand what to expect from the procedure. Second, they educate patients regarding potential adverse events and possible complications from procedures. Third, they educate patients regarding potential medications and activities that may compromise the postprocedure period or even the cosmetic out-come of the procedure. Finally, they allow the physi-cian to instruct the patient in the management of simple and common postprocedure issues and events that may occur.

In order for these instructions to be of the most benefit, it is essential that they be written in layman's terms. Instructions with complex medical terminol-ogy will only serve to confuse the patient, increase their anxiety regarding the procedure, and decrease their likelihood of achieving their desired outcome. The instructions should always be reviewed prior to the procedure with the patient. Ideally, once a patient decides to undergo a soft tissue filler aug-mentation, the pre- and postprocedure instructions should be reviewed in detail by the treating physician or an experienced member of the office team. It is not simply enough to hand over the instructions to the patient; rather, they should be reviewed and thor-oughly explained in a step-by-step manner. Patients should then be provided a written copy of these instructions to take home with them for their review.

Finally, on the instructions, there should be a clearly marked telephone number to the physician's office for the patient to call in the event of any confusion or further questions. The few minutes that the physician spends reviewing these instructions will help to forge a strong therapeutic alliance between the physician and the patient, allay the fears of the patient, and ultimately help the patient to achieve his or her desired realistic cosmetic outcome.

PREPROCEDURE INSTRUCTIONS

General Principles

Effective preprocedure instructions help prepare the patient by describing the technique, as well as setting the patient's expectations for the degree of improvement they should anticipate. Ideally, these points are discussed by the treating physician at the initial consultation, as well as during the process of informed consent. However, the preprocedure instructions should again reiterate these ideas. The instructions often contain information about the duration of the procedure, as well as the likely duration of the cosmetic effect. The instructions should also discuss the likelihood of bruising, as well as specific medications and activities that increase this risk. Patients should be informed about topical anesthetics, as well as the potential use of injected local anesthetics in the form of nerve blocks. Finally, the preprocedure instructions should discuss pain control, as well as products that could potentially help minimize swelling and facilitate more rapid achievement of the desired cosmetic improvement.

Medications to Avoid Prior to the Procedure

The preprocedure instructions should discuss the patient's activities, particularly focusing on their use of medications, in the days prior to undergoing their augmentation. Patients are now typically on multiple medications, both over the counter (OTC) and prescription, which can increase their risk of bruising. During the initial consultation, it is important for the physician to review and discuss all of the patient's prescription medications, OTC remedies, and herbal/vitamin supplements (including herbal teas) to determine whether the patient is taking anything regularly that is known to exacerbate bruising and swelling. These medications and supplements should be discontinued prior to the procedure, if possible, to make the process a more predictable and desirable experience.

Many patients are on aspirin, nonsteroidal anti-inflammatory drugs (NSAIDs), or other anticoagulants for a variety of reasons. Patients should be warned that these agents thin the blood and increase the risk of bruising and significant swelling associated with these procedures. Ideally, patients are instructed to avoid these agents for seven days prior to, as well as four to five days after, the procedure to decrease the risk of significant bruising and swelling. However, the decision as to whether to discontinue the medication depends on weighing the associated risks and benefits; clearly, these risks and benefits depend on the indication for the use of the anticoagulant.

In regard to *therapeutic* use of known anticoagulants, such as in patients with a history of a heart attack, stroke, or blood clot, it is our practice to keep these patients on these necessary medications. This clearly applies to patients on Coumadin, Plavix, as well as *therapeutic* aspirin. In cases where patients may suggest discontinuation of their own *therapeutic* anticoagulation, we discourage this and very carefully explain the potential risks associated with these patients being ineffectively anticoagulated far outweighs the benefit of decreased risk of bruising.[1,2] In addition, we encourage the patient to discuss these potential ramifications with their primary care physician, cardiologist, or neurologist and to be sure and explain to their physician that we will be performing an elective aesthetic treatment consisting of injections of a filler substance.

If patients are simply on aspirin for theoretic *preventative* measures (such as a family history of coronary artery disease), we usually have these patients discontinue their aspirin therapy at least seven days prior to the procedure. Finally, if patients routinely ingest aspirin or other NSAIDs for headache, muscle aches, and minor pain, we encourage these patients to discontinue at least seven days prior to the procedure. We indicate that as an alternative analgesic to aspirin and NSAIDs, acetaminophen (which will not affect coagulation) *can be used* for headaches and pain.

Aspirin results in *irreversible* inhibition of platelets through an irreversible inhibition of cyclooxygenase; as a result, aspirin continues to exert its effect after it is discontinued until new functional platelets are formed, which typically requires five or more days. Other NSAIDs (such as ibuprofen) *reversibly* inhibit platelet aggregation. Thus, the duration of their effect is determined by the half-life of the drug, which is typically a few hours, rather than the time necessary for platelets to regenerate. Theoretically, the increased risk of bruising associated with the use of reversible platelet inhibitors should decrease within a day or two (four to five half-lives) after the medication is discontinued. In practice, if antiplatelet agents are going to be discontinued for the procedure, we recommend that all antiplatelet agents and anticoagulants be stopped one week prior to the procedure to decrease the risk of significant bruising and swelling after the procedure.

Many herbal medications and vitamins have an inhibitory effect on platelets or other aspects of coagulation and therefore should also be avoided due to their increased risk of bruising. Manufacturers of herbal remedies are currently not required to submit efficacy or safety data to the US Food and Drug Administration (FDA). As a result, the beneficial effects and side effects of these herbal remedies are not well characterized; furthermore, the manufacturers are not required to print these potential

adverse effects on their labeling. Patients must be instructed regarding the potential increased risk of bleeding/bruising associated with several specific herbal medications. We typically list the following supplements and suggest that they be avoided for at least one week prior to the treatment: garlic (*Allium sativum* L.), ginger (*Zingiber officinale* Roscoe), ginseng (*Panax ginseng* CA Meyer and *Panax quinquefloius* L.), gingko biloba (*Gingko biloba* L.), kava (*Piper methysticum*), celery root (*Apium graveolens* Rapaceum Group), fish oils (Omega-3 fatty acids), St. John's wort (*Hypericum perforatum* L.), vitamin E (at higher doses in the range of 1,000–2,000 IU per day), and glucosamine/chondroitin. The patient should also avoid these medications for four to five days postprocedure as well, especially if bruising is visible within one to two days after the procedure. A more comprehensive list of supplements and other agents known to have an anticoagulant effect has been published in two recent articles.[3,4]

Finally, moderate doses of alcohol have been reported to result in reduced morbidity from coronary heart disease; this is thought to occur by the inhibition of platelet activation, although the exact mechanism is not well characterized.[5] Although this inhibition of platelet activation is of benefit in reducing coronary heart disease risk, its use in the periprocedure period increases the risk of bruising and swelling following soft tissue filler augmentation. Clotting factors are clearly made in the liver, but some of the effect of alcohol may also be due to simple vasodilation as well. Thus, typically we advise our patients to avoid alcohol for at least five days prior to the procedure and at least the first two to three days after the procedure.

Medications that May Be of Benefit in Reducing Bruising

Although the majority of our discussion regarding medications focuses on those that increase the risk of bruising, there have been promising reports of agents that may decrease the risk of bruising and swelling associated with procedures. Although it is ultimately at the discretion of each individual physician as to whether or not to advocate the use of these substances, it is important that physicians be familiar with these reports.

Arnica, *Arnica montana*, both topical and oral, has previously been anecdotally reported to result in decreased bruising in patients undergoing procedures. A recent randomized, double-blind, placebo-controlled clinical trial compared patients undergoing rhytidectomy, treated with either oral placebo or oral arnica three times daily for four days beginning the morning of surgery. Arnica-treated patients developed statistically significant smaller areas of ecchymosis after the procedure. However, no objective difference in the degree of ecchymosis as assessed by the extent of color change nor any subjective improvements noted by either the physicians or the patients were determined in the study.[6] Thus, it is not completely clear as to whether or not the arnica was truly of any significant benefit in this study. It is therefore at the discretion of the treating physician as to whether or not to recommend periprocedure oral arnica.

Bromelain is the name given to a family of proteolytic enzymes derived from the pineapple plant, *Ananas comosus*. It has been reported to result in reduced edema, bruising, pain, and healing time after trauma and surgical procedures. Unfortunately, the majority of these studies were performed in the 1960s and 1970s, and subsequently, there have been conflicting results among studies. One study of 53 patients undergoing rhinoplasty revealed decreased swelling and ecchymosis associated with bromelain use;[7] however, a further study of 154 plastic surgery patients demonstrated no statistically significant difference in edema between the bromelain and placebo groups.[8] Bromelain has also been reported to increase the rate of resorption of postprocedure

hematomas, if given at the time of hematoma injection and for the next week.[9] Unfortunately, bromelain has also been reported to prevent aggregation of platelets in patients with high platelet aggregation values; it is not clear whether this same inhibition occurs in the healthy normal population.[10] Thus, given this ambiguity, as well as the fact that the majority of the scientific studies are forty years old, it is difficult to determine with certainty whether bromelain in the periprocedure period is of any benefit.

Finally, topical vitamin K may be of benefit in reducing the bruising associated with soft tissue augmentation. A recent randomized, double-blind study demonstrated that topical vitamin K applied twice daily for two weeks after pulse dye laser treatment reduced the severity of bruising associated with the procedure.[11] However, other studies have demonstrated no significant reduction in bruising associated with the use of topical vitamin K. Again, the ultimate decision resides with each physician as to whether to recommend the use of topical vitamin K in the periprocedure period.

DAY OF PROCEDURE INSTRUCTIONS

Duration and Extent of Procedure

One of the major draws of injectable fillers for cosmetic patients is that it is a minimally invasive, rapid procedure that results in an obvious immediate cosmetic improvement. Although it is true that the actual injection of the filler may be relatively quick, patients should be informed that the entire visit might take longer, particularly if the physician is utilizing topical anesthesia. In this type of circumstance, time can ideally be utilized to review the procedure, obtain informed consent, and photograph the patient to establish their preprocedure appearance. By establishing the likely duration of the visit prior to the patient arriving, their level of anxiety and overall experience will be improved.

Makeup

Patients should be instructed not to wear any makeup to the office within the proposed treatment area on the day of the procedure. It is important that preprocedure photographs are taken of the patient's natural appearance to demonstrate the full effect of the soft tissue augmentation. If patients are wearing makeup, this should be removed completely prior to photography and administering the injections. The concern is that the makeup may make it difficult to appropriately prep the skin or could potentially result in implantation of the makeup material in the skin. This potential for implantation of foreign material could have possibly been a factor in some rare reports of adverse events such as abscesses, possible biofilm infections, or foreign body giant cell reactions after dermal filler implantation.[19]

Additionally, though many might consider this overkill, we actually instruct the patient not to apply any makeup to the treated area until the morning after the procedure. Our rationale is that the puncture sites in the skin are not healed immediately after the injections, and applied makeup may cause blockage or even increase the risk of infection of these sites as the patient's makeup itself or fingertips may not be completely clean. If your facility or the patient has new or clean makeup and the application is very clean (cotton tip applicator or at least washed hands), this may not be necessary especially when using smaller gauge needles.

Anesthesia

Filler injections are minimally invasive; however, providing or offering different forms of anesthesia is important in ensuring that patients have the best possible experience. Anesthesia can be adequately achieved via either topical anesthesia or regional anesthesia with nerve blocks. Ultimately, it is at the discretion of the treating physician as to whether the topical or regional anesthesia will be used, but we recommend having the patient be a coparticipant in this decision-making process.

It is important to keep in mind that if topical anesthesia is to be used, patients must be aware of the need for application prior to the procedure. We typically recommend OTC LMX (4 percent lidocaine; Ferndale Labs, Ferndale, MI) or prescription EMLA (Eutectic Mixture of Local Anesthetics; Abraxis Pharmaceutical Products, Schaumburg, IL) to be applied at the sites of filler injection one hour prior to the procedure, as well as a reapplication thirty minutes prior to the procedure. We recommend covering the topical anesthetic with cellophane wrap to increase penetration and overall efficacy. We explain very carefully to have patients apply the anesthetic only to the areas being treated (such as nasolabial folds, oral commissures, and mid-cheek). In addition, we do not have patients schedule other procedures requiring topical anesthesia for the same day. Keep in mind that there have been reports of lidocaine toxicity when using high concentration compounded topical anesthetic agents applied to large surface areas (and often under occlusion) such as prior to laser hair removal. In addition, we screen patients for a history of sulfa allergy as many topical formulations contain Ester anesthetic derivatives, which contain a sulfa moiety, and thus, the potential for cross-reactivity exists. For this reason as well, we often favor a noncompounded lidocaine formulation alone or in combination with other members of the Amide family of anesthetics. Many physicians feel that compounded higher concentration products convey a better anesthetic effect, such as compounded BLT (benzocaine, lidocaine, tetracaine). In addition, a topical anesthetic occlusive mask has been FDA approved containing lidocaine and tetracaine (Pliaglis; ZARS Pharma, Salt Lake City, UT), which is applied as a cream and dries as a mask, thereby offering some occlusive properties.

Regional nerve blocks can also be used to achieve adequate anesthesia. A full discussion of nerve blocks, the relevant anatomy, and injection technique is given in other sections. In our experience, nerve blocks are often not necessary if adequate topical anesthesia is utilized for most areas, with the exception of lip augmentation. If regional anesthesia is to be used, patients should be informed prior to the procedure that the anesthetized area will have decreased feeling for up to a couple of hours. This can be problematic if the patient manipulates the area, as they will likely not be able to judge the strength of the manipulation as well as any resulting adverse effects, such as biting the corner of their mouth. Additionally, patients should be cautioned to avoid extremely hot or cold beverages after the procedure, as sensation will be impaired until the anesthesia wears off. For lip augmentation, often a mini-block or sulcus block can be used to create a ring block of the area of the mouth and isolate the area of anesthesia. In addition, short-acting more traditional dental anesthetics, such as articaine, can be used to quicken the resolution of the anesthetic effect to about one hour.

Activities

It is our practice to instruct patients to avoid exercise on the day of the procedure, as this can lead to increased swelling. Additionally, although many patients choose soft tissue augmentation because of its lack of significant downtime compared to surgical procedures, we encourage them not to schedule *important* social events for seven to ten days following the procedure. This is to ensure that if the patient does develop significant swelling or bruising associated with the procedure, they have sufficient time to recover prior to their event. Again, if this is emphasized to the patient prior to having the procedure performed, the patient will have more appropriate expectations and hopefully avoid potentially problematic times on their social or work calendars.

Pre- and Postprocedure Photographs

Detailed pre- and postprocedure photographs should be taken both to document the clinical improvement for the physician's chart records and to demonstrate the improvement to the patient. Ideally, these photographs should be taken by the same camera, in the same orientation, and in the same lighting to reduce any other variables; however, in practice, a handheld digital camera is typically adequate. To further establish the degree of improvement, pictures can be taken *during* the course of the procedure to document improvement in a treated area versus a nontreated area. For instance, if patients are having their bilateral nasolabial fold creases augmented, a photograph can be taken after one nasolabial fold is augmented. This photograph demonstrates the full improvement associated with the procedure and is often easier for the patient to note the change compared to the untreated side. These photographs are particularly important if patients later feel that they did not achieve their desired outcome or are unsatisfied.

Postprocedure Instructions

Swelling and Bruising

Immediately after the procedure, the most commonly reported side effects are temporary redness and swelling at the injection sites. As these are likely to happen in all patients to some degree, it is important to address these issues in the postprocedure instructions. It is important to emphasize that this swelling and redness is temporary and will often resolve in the first two to three days after the procedure.

Bruising is also a common postprocedure side effect (Figure 15.1). Patients should again be reminded that certain medications, OTC analgesics, and herbal remedies can thin the blood and thereby increase the risk of bruising. A complete discussion of these medications can be found in the preprocedure instructions. Patients are instructed to avoid medications that thin

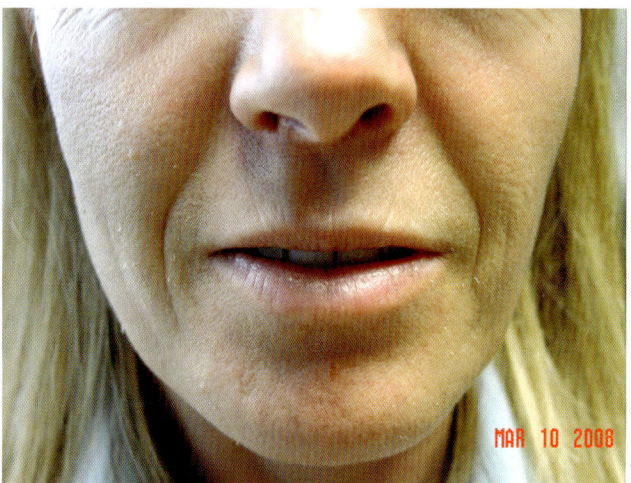 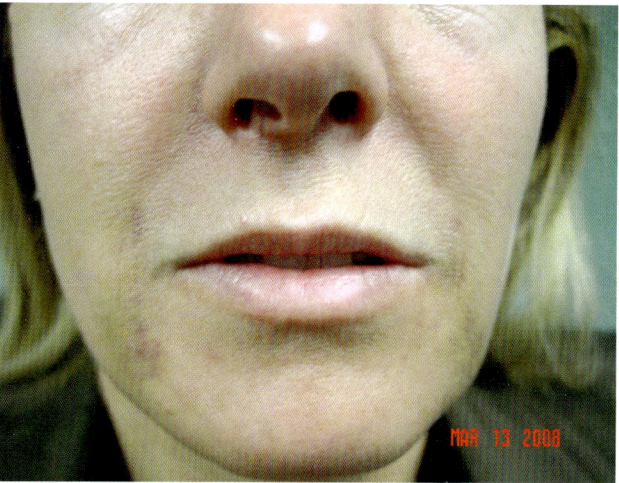

FIG. 15.1. *Pre- and Posttreatment with hyaluronic acid in the nasolabial folds and oral commissures. Note moderate amount of bruising three days posttreatment with a nice correction.*

the blood for five to seven days after the procedure, especially if some bruising is apparent by two days following the procedure in order to decrease the risk of accentuating the bruising. Additionally, we recommend that patients avoid alcohol consumption for a day or two after the procedure due to the theoretical increased risk of bruising as well.

Cold compresses applied immediately to injection sites after the procedure can also help decrease the potential swelling and bruising. We therefore instruct patients to apply cold compresses, in the form of gel packs, frozen peas, or even sandwich bags filled with ice cubes, three to four times a day for twenty minutes at a time. Usually, we encourage patients to stay in the office for the initial icing immediately after the procedure, so as to minimize swelling and bruising from the outset. They are instructed to continue these cold compresses for two and sometimes three days after the procedure. We do not typically recommend these cold compresses to the glabella, as this cold-induced vasoconstriction could theoretically increase the risk of necrosis in this area of watershed blood supply.

If a patient has very significant bruising two to three days after a filler procedure, some experienced physicians have found that using a pulse dye laser is helpful in expediting the resolution of the bruising. We reserve this for those patients who are very concerned about the bruising and might have an unanticipated social event quickly approaching. Again anecdotally, the pulse dye laser is used focally over the significant bruise with consideration to settings in the area of 7.5 Joules and 6 milliseconds with a 10-mm spot size.

Necrosis

Skin necrosis is an extremely rare adverse event associated with the use of injectable fillers. It is typically a result of interruption of the vascular supply to the area by compression, obstruction of the vessel(s) with filler material, and/or direct injury to the vessel(s).[12] Although this typically occurs rapidly after injection, there have been cases of necrosis developing several hours after injection. Thus, although postprocedure instructions do not usually need to discuss skin necrosis in detail as it is indeed unlikely, there should be a brief note stating that if patients begin to observe blue or black discoloration of the skin or suffer from extreme pain or progressive increasing pain, they should call the treating

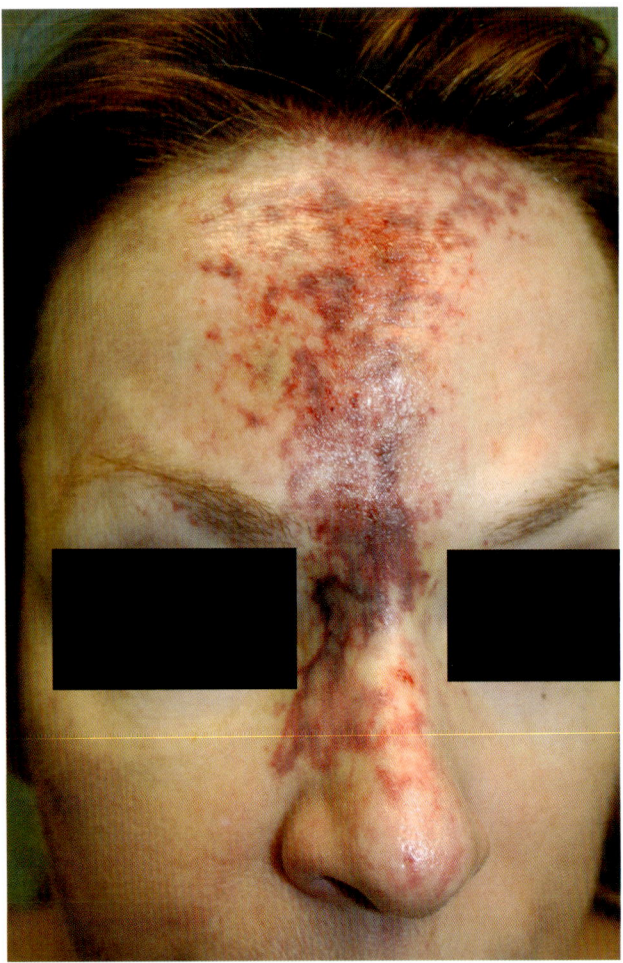

FIG. 15.2. *Violaceous reticulated pattern of impending necrosis 14 hours after an injection of hyaluronic acid filler in the glabella. (Reprinted with permission from J Cohen, M Brown. Anatomic Considerations for Soft Tissue Augmentation of the Face. Journal of Drugs in Dermatology, Jan 2009; 8(1), 13–16.)*

physician immediately (Figure 15.2). This is extremely important, as there has recently been published a treatment algorithm with hyaluronidase for impending necrosis;[13] obviously, earlier treatment with hyaluronidase resulting in reestablishing vascular flow would potentially result in less necrosis and an improved patient outcome if the filler used was a hyaluronic acid derivative.

Manipulation of the Area After Procedure

Patients are often very tempted to touch and manipulate the augmented area after the procedure. This is problematic for several reasons: First of all, the area is still anesthetized, and as a result, the patients may not realize the degree to which they are manipulating the product. Second, excessive manipulation may increase the risk of swelling or bruising associated with the procedure. Finally, manipulation could cause migration of the product, thereby compromising the patient's cosmetic outcome. Thus, we recommend that the patients avoid touching, cleaning, or manipulating the augmented areas for the first few hours after treatment.

The day after the procedure, the patient can touch and massage the area gently. If the patient begins to notice early nodule formation or accumulation of product, they can gently massage the area. However, if the accumulation or nodule persists, we would prefer that the patient return to the office for evaluation rather than continuing to manipulate the area themselves. Thus, postprocedure instructions state that the patient should also call the office if they notice nodule formation after the procedure. This allows the treating physician to correct the imperfection and allows for the best possible cosmetic outcome for the patient.

Follow-Up

Immediate routine follow-up after the procedure is not necessary in our opinion. However, for patients who are extremely concerned about their outcome or for those who develop immediate bruising after the procedure, follow-up in five to seven days can be particularly comforting. This allows adequate time for the swelling and bruising to decrease and allows for the treating physician to observe the full benefit of the procedure. At this time, subtle touch-up injections can be given if needed. A few of the currently marketed fillers are available in smaller sizes, which are particularly useful for touch-ups.

Patients should also very clearly be informed, both verbally and in writing on the procedure consent form, that if they have a temporary filler (such as hyaluronic acid or collagen), the degree of augmentation will decrease after several months. Depending on the filler product, physicians may choose to schedule these patients for a follow-up visit in four to six months to assess the remaining effect of the soft tissue augmentation, as well as schedule the patient for further filler injections if so desired.

SPECIAL CIRCUMSTANCES

Antiviral Prophylaxis

Herpes simplex virus type 1 (HSV-1) is a common infection of the oral area; up to 30 percent of patients will experience chronic outbreaks of HSV-1 from reactivation of latent infection in a nerve ganglion. This reactivation can be stimulated by trauma, surgery, or other procedural interventions (Figure 15.3). Several small case series and studies have demonstrated that prophylaxis with acyclovir or valacyclovir prior to invasive procedures, particularly laser resurfacing, reduces the risk of reactivation of HSV-1 infections.

There is potential that the injection of soft tissue fillers may be sufficiently traumatic to cause recurrent herpes simplex outbreaks in susceptible patients. Unfortunately, to date, there are no large trials determining the exact risk or likelihood of reactivation of HSV-1 infections in patients undergoing soft tissue augmentation with fillers. Given the lack of morbidity associated with prophylaxis, as well as the potential to reactivate latent HSV-1 infections, we recommend that patients with a history of oral herpes simplex infections be treated with antiviral prophylaxis prior to undergoing lip augmentation.

There are multiple antiviral treatment regimens depending on whether the patient is immunocompromised or not. A recent study of immunocompetent patients undergoing laser skin resurfacing demonstrated that oral valacyclovir 500 mg dosed twice daily, beginning the day prior to the procedure,

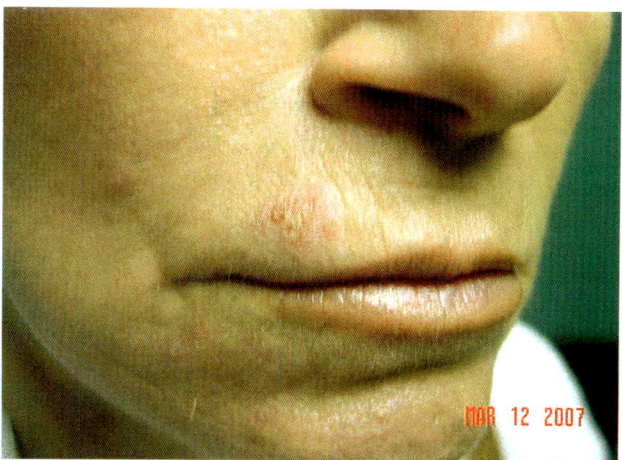

FIG. 15.3. *Reactivation of herpes simplex virus resulting in a cold sore few days after a nonablative fractionated laser was used on the upper lip.*

and continuing for ten days was as effective as a 500 mg twice daily for fourteen days at HSV-1 prophylaxis.[14] Although this is a laser study and not directly related to soft tissue augmentation with fillers, there are unfortunately no direct data to establish the ideal dosing or duration of antiviral prophylaxis in soft tissue augmentation procedures. Thus, these represent the best available data at this time. We typically prescribe valacyclovir 500 mg orally twice a day to our patients with a history of HSV; the prophylaxis is to begin typically a day or two prior to the lip augmentation procedure, and the patients complete a five- to seven- day course. Aside from injecting the lips themselves, we do not typically give patients any prophylaxis for other common areas of filler injections such as the nasolabial folds or oral commissures. Ultimately, as there are no definitive data on the utility or the duration of antiviral prophylaxis, this decision as to whether to prophylax as well as the treatment regimen rests with the treating physician.

Previous Use of Oral Retinoids

A number of current cosmetic patients have previously undergone treatment with isotretinoin, a systemic retinoid, for severe nodulocystic acne. Although these treatments are generally well tolerated by the patients, there have been reports of impaired wound healing and keloid formation as a result of systemic retinoid therapy. A total of nine cases have been described detailing keloidal scarring after dermabrasion in patients either currently or previously treated with oral isotretinoin.[15,16] Interestingly, since that time, there have been numerous reports of successful dermabrasion procedures being performed on patients either recently or concurrently treated with isotretinoin, without the development of keloidal scarring. Additionally, animal model studies have demonstrated no significant impairment in wound healing as a result of isotretinoin use.[17] Thus, the potential adverse effect on scar formation and wound healing in patients previously treated with isotretinoin is unclear. However, the standard of care in laser resurfacing has evolved to include the avoidance of systemic retinoids in the perioperative period, especially within the six months prior to the procedure.

Though some physicians may feel this precaution could extend to the avoidance of systemic retinoids in the periprocedure period when performing soft tissue augmentation with filling agents, the authors feel this is most likely safe; however, we often wait three to six months after discontinuing the systemic retinoids prior to performing the augmentation if possible. This type of decision seems to arise more frequently in patients with significant acne scars who may have just completed a course of isotretinoin and now have a major social event such as a wedding. This decision, ultimately, is at the discretion of the treating physician due to the lack of definitive evidence.

Psychiatric Issues

As a result of the increased number of cosmetic procedures being performed in the United States, it is more likely that treating physicians will encounter patients undergoing procedures who are affected by some type of psychological issue. Body dysmorphic disorder is defined in the DSM IV criteria as "the patient is preoccupied with an imagined defect of appearance or is excessively concerned about a slight physical anomaly."[18] It is disproportionately encountered by physicians performing cosmetic procedures, as these patients often seek to change their perceived imperfections. Unfortunately, body dysmorphic disorder is frequently unrecognized or underdiagnosed by physicians. This becomes problematic, as lack of recognition of some of these signs can ultimately lead to greater difficulties for both the patient and the treating physician.

Unfortunately, as the perceived defect is often either absent or slight, the patient does not typically benefit greatly from cosmetic procedures. Very often, the patient continues to be preoccupied with the perceived deficiency and is dissatisfied with the treatment. In our experience, these patients make frequent phone calls to the office and prolonged visits after the procedure to review their pre- and post-procedure photographs; many of these patients after a reasonable discussion of the limitations of procedures or advice on psychological care will simply seek cosmetic treatment elsewhere. Body dysmorphic disorder has been reported to improve with cognitive-behavioral therapy, coupled with exposure therapy; it is not improved with further surgical intervention. It is imperative that the physicians performing cosmetic procedures be familiar with the signs and symptoms of body dysmorphic disorder, so that they can actively screen their patients. If a physician is concerned that one of their patients may have body dysmorphic disorder, this patient should be referred to a psychiatrist for diagnosis and treatment evaluation.

Unsatisfied Patients

It is a reality that although most patients undergoing soft tissue augmentation will be very pleased with their outcomes, there will always be a few patients who are unsatisfied with their postprocedure appearance. One of the most important ways to limit the number of unsatisfied patients is to set reasonable expectations for the procedure before the patient undergoes their augmentation. Pictures of patients previously treated with fillers are a great way to help the patient set realistic expectations. If after the procedure, patients are dissatisfied with their improvement, we recommend they come back to the office for a follow-up visit. This visit allows a specific comparison of the patient's pre- and postprocedure pictures, so that both the physician and the patient can then analyze the cosmetic outcome. This will help to facilitate an honest discussion of the patient's desired outcome, degree of improvement already achieved, and what is realistic to be able to achieve with additional procedures. This is an essential component of building a strong doctor–patient relationship and is important in obtaining a very satisfied cosmetic patient who might be interested in scheduling additional cosmetic procedures.

CONCLUSIONS

Minimally invasive cosmetic procedures have exploded in popularity in the last few years; these procedures are desired by the public not only for their dramatic improvement in appearance but also for the rapidity and lack of significant downtime associated with the procedure. However, that is not to say that these procedures should be taken lightly or minimized by either the patient or the physician.

Effectively written patient instructions can play a very key role in the success of a cosmetic physician. These instructions can help to explain the procedure, as well as set the patient's expectations. Furthermore, these instructions should list medications to be avoided in the pre- and postprocedure period to help patients achieve their ideal cosmetic outcome. Finally, the instructions should discuss common questions regarding activities and care of the augmented sites after the procedure. These instructions ultimately not only save time and effort for the physician, but more importantly, they also empower and educate patients to help them achieve their ideal cosmetic outcome.

REFERENCES

1. Otley CC. Perioperative evaluation and management in dermatologic surgery. *J Am Acad Dermatol* 2006 Jan; **54**(1):119–127.

2. Schanbacher CF, Bennett RG. Postoperative stroke after stopping warfarin for cutaneous surgery. *Dermatol Surg* 2000 Aug;**26**(8):785–789.

3. Dinehart SM, Henry L. Dietary supplements: altered coagulation and effects on bruising. *Dermatol Surg* 2005 Jul;**31**(7 Pt 2):819–826; discussion 826.

4. Collins SC, Dufresne RG. Dietary supplements in the setting of mohs surgery. *Dermatol Surg* 2002 Jun; **28**(6):447–452.

5. Kasuda S, Sakurai Y, Shima M, et al. Inhibition of PAR4 signaling mediates ethanol-induced attenuation of platelet function in vitro. *Alcohol Clin Exp Res* 2006;**30**(9):1608–1614.

6. Seeley BM, Denton AB, Ahn MS, et al. Effect of homeopathic Arnica montana on bruising in face-lifts: results of a randomized, double-blind, placebo-controlled clinical trial. *Arch Facial Plast Surg* 2006;**8**(1):54–59.

7. Seltzer AP. Minimizing post-operative edema and ecchymoses by the use of an oral enzyme preparation (bromelain). A controlled study of 53 rhinoplasty cases. *Eye Ear Nose Throat Mon* 1962;**41**:813–817.

8. Gylling U, Rintala A, Taipale S, et al. The effect of a proteolytic enzyme combinate (bromelain) on the postoperative oedema by oral application. A clinical and experimental study. *Acta Chir Scand* 1966;**131**(3): 193–196.

9. Woolf RM, Snow JW, Walker JH, et al. Resolution of an artificially induced hematoma and the influence of a proteolytic enzyme. *J Trauma* 1965;**83**:491–494.

10. MacKay D, Miller AL. Nutritional support for wound healing. *Altern Med Rev* 2003;**8**(4):359–377.

11. Shah NS, Lazarus MC, Bugdodel R, et al. The effects of topical vitamin K on bruising after laser treatment. *J Am Acad Dermatol* 2004;**50**(6):982–983.

12. Hanke CW, Higley HR, Jolivette DM, et al. Abscess formation and local necrosis after treatment with Zyderm or Zyplast collagen implant. *J Am Acad Dermatol* 1991;**25**:319–326.

13. Hirsch RJ, Cohen JL, Carruthers JD. Successful management of an unusual presentation of impending necrosis following a hyaluronic acid injection embolus and a proposed algorithm for management with hyaluronidase. *Dermatol Surg* 2007;**33**(3):357–360.

14. Beeson WH, Rachel JD. Valacyclovir prophylaxis for herpes simplex virus infection or infection recurrence following laser skin resurfacing. *Dermatol Surg* 2002;**28**(4):331–336.

15. Rubenstein R, Roenigk HH Jr, Stegman SJ, et al. Atypical keloids after dermabrasion of patients taking isotretinoin. *J Am Acad Dermatol* 1986;**15**(2 Pt 1):280–285.

16. Zachariae H. Delayed wound healing and keloid formation following argon laser treatment or dermabrasion during isotretinoin treatment. *Br J Dermatol* 1988;**118**(5):703–706.

17. Moy RL, Moy LS, Bennett RG, Zitelli JA, Uitto J. Systemic isotretinoin: effects on dermal wound healing in a rabbit ear model in vivo. *J Dermatol Surg Oncol* 1990 Dec;**16**(12):1142–1146.

18. American Psychiatric Association (ed.). Diagnostic and Statistical Manual of Mental Disorders. Fourth Edition, *Text Revised (DSM-IV)*. Washington, DC: American Psychiatric Association; 2000.

19. Narins RS, Jewell M, Rubin M, Cohen JL, et al. Clinical conference: management of rare events following dermal fillers – focal necrosis and angry red bumps. *Dermatol Surg* 2006;**32**:426–434.

Chapter 16

CONCLUSION: FUTURE TRENDS IN FILLERS

by

Neil S. Sadick, MD

The present treatise has outlined the major advances in the development and utilization of fillers in the United States. Fillers are playing an ever-expanding role within this clinical setting. Combination programs employing toxins, fillers, light source, and radiofrequency technologies make up the backbone of noninvasive photorejuvenation programs. The therapeutic armentarium of fillers available in this country continues to evolve annually. There are six major trends in next-generation fillers that have evolved in this regard. A well-accepted and standardized classification schema of these agents has yet to be evolved.

LONGER ACTING FILLING AGENTS

There is definitely a trend toward longer acting fillers. In our busy world and for economic reasons, individuals would like to minimize the number of filler treatments that are necessary while still maintaining effect. The major question that is not universally accepted is what is that optimal duration of effect? Most physicians feel that an intermediate-acting filler with duration of twelve to eighteen months is

optimal.[1] This allows for longevity greater than older generation collagens and traditional hyaluronic acid derivatives; however, if there are adverse sequelae, it will resolve within a reasonable period of time, although one may expect as we move down the road that this timeline may continue to expand.

SITE-SPECIFIC FILLERS

Another major trend in fillers is specific capabilities. This means that they have clinical and physical characteristics that are uniquely beneficial for given anatomic areas. Examples of such site-specific areas are the lips and tear troughs, where lighter fillers with greater laminar flow characteristics would be more beneficial.[2] Examples of such fillers are Evolence Breeze and Restylane Fine Line. Market demand will encourage aesthetic companies to develop fillers that will differentiate them in this ever increasingly competitive arena.

VOLUMIZERS

A recent trend in pan-facial augmentation is volumetric repletion. As we achieve a greater understanding of photoaging, we have come to understand that it is not just about lines and wrinkles but rather about volume loss involving the entire facial structural anatomy not only at the level of the dermis but involving deeper structures including fat, muscle, and bone as well.[3] In this stead, newer generation fillers have recently been introduced that address these needs. Let the reader not forget that autologous fat remains the gold standard for facial volume replacement.[4] As a further developmental milestone, poly-L-lactic acid was introduced as a pan-facial volume repletion agent initially for management of HIV lipoatrophy and subsequently for aesthetic rejuvenation.[5] As time progressed, other products such as calcium hydroxylapatite (Radiesse), Perlane, and Juvederm Ultra Plus were introduced to fill the niche of localized volume augmentation.[6]

Newer generation products such as Voluma and Restylane SubQ are presently in global clinical trials and may be available in the United States at some point in the near future. This trend is certainly one that is being increasingly recognized as one of the major future trends in filler development.

BIOACTIVE AGENTS

One of the mechanisms of longevity action claims being purported by manufacturers is through the mechanism of biostimulation. This has been particularly elaborated upon for the larger molecular weight fillers. These claims state that implantation of foreign filler agents can induce a dermal remodeling response similar to what we see with dermal heating produced by laser and radiofrequency sources.[7] Ultrastructural studies have shown fibroblast activation and new collagen synthesis in this regard.[8,9] In addition, epidermal thickening has been claimed but has not been well substantiated in this setting. These claims have been made for large

molecular fillers such as poly-L-acid (Sculptra) and calcium hydroxylapatite (Radiesse).

In addition, other filler agents such as Restylane have been reported in the literature to induce dermal remodeling with new collagen synthesis by means of tissue stretching with viscous mechanical properties leading to subsequent neocollagenesis.[10]

The major question to be answered is how much long-term effect is secondary to the filler itself and how much is due to actual dermal remodeling effect. The problem in the literature is that most of the studies that are reported to date are short-term studies. Ongoing, long-term studies using several large molecular agents are now in progress. Hopefully, these studies will provide answers to these questions in the near future.

WHOLE-BODY REJUVENATION PRODUCTS

If one were to look into a crystal ball into the near future, one would almost certainly see the greater utilization and new development of fillers for whole-body rejuvenation. We are already seeing an increasing number of patients being treated for hand volume augmentation with calcium hydroxylapatite (Radiesse) and poly-L-lactic (Sculptra). Other pioneering off-face potential cellulite treatment areas include the décolleté, cellulite areas of depression, and postliposuction defects.

HYBRID PRODUCTS

As we move down the road of new technologies, we will see the evolution of many new approaches in the development of novel filler products. Combinations of collagen or hyaluronic acid plus calcium hydroxylapatite are already being explored. Synergistic effects of multiple compounded products would explain the potential rationale of this approach.

In conclusion, it is an exciting time in the filler world. The aesthetic physician is faced with many valuable treatment options for their patients. Stay tuned as the world is constantly changing and the quest for the optimal filler continues to evolve.

REFERENCES

1. Goldman MP. Optimizing the use of fillers for facial rejuvenation: the right tool for the right job. *Cosmet Dermatol.* 2007; **20**(7): S3 14–25.

2. Sadick NS. Soft tissue augmentation: selection, mode of operation and proper use of injectable agents. *Cosmet Dermatol.* 2007; **20**(5): S2 8–13.

3. Sadick NS, Karcher C, Palmisano L. Cosmetic dermatology of the aging face. *Clin Dermatol.* 2009 (in press).

4. Kaufman MR, Miller TA, et al. Autologous fat transfer for facial recontouring: is there science behind the art? *Plast Reconst Surg.* 2007; **119**: 2287–2296.

5. Vleggaar D. Facial volumetric correction with injectable poly-L-lactic acid. *Dermatol Surg.* 2005; **31**: 1511–1518.

6. Dayan SH. Bassichis BA. Facial dermal fillers: selection of appropriate products and techniques. *Aesthet Surg J.* 2008; **28**: 335–347.

7. Keni SP, Sidle DM. Sculptra (injectable poly-L-lactic acid). *Facial Plast Surg.* 2007; **15**: 91–97.

8. Wang F. Garza LA, et al. In vivo stimulation of de novo collagen production caused by cross-linked hyaluronic acid dermal filler injected into photodamaged human skin. *Arch Dermatol.* 2007; **143**: 155–163.

9. Holzapfel A, Mangat D, Barron D. Soft-tissue augmentation with calcium hydroxylapatite. *Arch Facial Plast Surg.* 2008; **10**: 335–338.

10. Solakoglu S, Tiryaki T, Ciloglu SE. The effect of cultured autologous fibroblasts on longevity of cross-linked hyaluronic acid used as a filler. *Aesthet Surg J.* 2008; **28**: 412–416.

Index